Current Management of Lesser Toe Disorders

Guest Editor

JOHN T. CAMPBELL, MD

FOOT AND ANKLE CLINICS

www.foot.theclinics.com

Consulting Editor
MARK S. MYERSON, MD

December 2011 • Volume 16 • Number 4

SAUNDERS an imprint of ELSEVIER, Inc.

W.B. SAUNDERS COMPANY
A Division of Elsevier Inc.

1600 John F. Kennedy Blvd. • Suite 1800 • Philadelphia, PA 19103-2899

http://www.theclinics.com

FOOT AND ANKLE CLINICS Volume 16, Number 4
December 2011 ISSN 1083-7515, ISBN-13: 978-1-4557-0449-1

Editor: David Parsons
Developmental Editor: Donald Mumford

Foot and Ankle Clinics (ISSN 1083-7515) is published quarterly by Elsevier, Inc., 360 Park Avenue South, New York, NY 10010-1710. Months of issue are March, June, September, and December. Periodicals postage paid at New York, NY, and additional mailing offices. Subscription price per year is $295.00 (US individuals), $386.00 (US institutions), $146.00 (US students), $336.00 (Canadian individuals), $456.00 (Canadian institutions), $201.00 (Canadian students), $433.00 (foreign individuals), $556.00 (foreign institutions), and $201.00 (foreign students). To receive student/resident rate, orders must be accompanied by name of affiliated institution, date of term, and the signature of program/residency coordinator on institution letterhead. Orders will be billed at individual rate until proof of status is received. Foreign air speed delivery is included in all *Clinics* subscription prices. All prices are subject to change without notice. **POSTMASTER:** Send address changes to *Foot and Ankle Clinics,* Elsevier Health Sciences Division, Subscription Customer Service, 3251 Riverport Lane, Maryland Heights, MO 63043. **Customer Service: 1-800-654-2452 (US and Canada). From outside of the United States and Canada, call 314-447-8871. Fax: 314-447-8029. E-mail: JournalsCustomerService-usa@elsevier.com (for print support); JournalsOnlineSupport-usa@elsevier.com (for online support).**

Reprints. For copies of 100 or more, of articles in this publication, please contact the Commercial Reprints Department, Elsevier Inc., 360 Park Avenue South, New York, NY 10010-1710. Tel.: 212-633-3812; Fax: 212-462-1935; E-mail: reprints@elsevier.com.

Printed and bound by CPI Group (UK) Ltd, Croydon, CR0 4YY

Transferred to Digital Print 2011

Contributors

CONSULTING EDITOR

MARK S. MYERSON, MD
Director, Institute for Foot and Ankle Reconstruction at Mercy, Mercy Medical Center, Baltimore, Maryland

GUEST EDITOR

JOHN T. CAMPBELL, MD
Institute for Foot and Ankle Reconstruction at Mercy, Mercy Medical Center, Baltimore, Maryland

AUTHORS

STEVEN ARNDT, MD
Foot and Ankle Fellow, Foot and Ankle Center, Orthopaedic and Rheumatologic Institute, Cleveland Clinic Main Campus, Cleveland, Ohio

TODD BERTRAND, MD
Resident, Orthopaedic Surgery, Department of Orthopaedic Surgery, Duke University School of Medicine, Durham, North Carolina

JAMES D. CALDER, MD, FRCS (Tr&Orth), FFSEM (UK)
Consultant Trauma and Orthopaedic Surgeon, Department of Orthopaedics, Chelsea and Westminster Hospital, London, United Kingdom

REBECCA A. CERRATO, MD
Institute for Foot and Ankle Reconstruction, Mercy Medical Center, Baltimore, Maryland

CAROLYN CHADWICK, MBChB, FRCSEd (Tr&Orth)
Foot and Ankle Fellow, Brisbane Foot and Ankle Centre, Brisbane Private Hospital, Brisbane, Australia

MARK S. DAVIES, FRCS Tr&Orth
London Foot and Ankle Centre, Hospital of St John and St Elizabeth, London, United Kingdom

RICHARD J. DE ASLA, MD
Chief, Foot & Ankle Division, Department of Orthopaedic Surgery, Massachusetts General Hospital; Clinical Instructor, Harvard Medical School, Boston, Massachusetts

J. KENT ELLINGTON, MD, MS
Foot and Ankle Institute, OrthoCarolina; Adjunct Assistant Professor of Biology, University of North Carolina—Charlotte; Faculty, Department of Orthopaedic Surgery, Carolinas Medical Center, Charlotte, North Carolina

JOHN Y. KWON, MD
Foot & Ankle Division, Department of Orthopaedic Surgery, Massachusetts General Hospital; Clinical Instructor, Harvard Medical School, Boston, Massachusetts

HO-SEONG LEE, MD
Professor of Medicine, Department of Orthopaedic Surgery, Asan Medical Center, College of Medicine, Ulsan University, Seoul, South Korea

WOO-CHUN LEE, MD
Professor of Medicine, Department of Orthopaedic Surgery, Seoul Paik Hospital, College of Medicine, Inje University, Seoul, South Korea

ANDREW MOLLOY, FRCS Tr&Orth
Consultant Orthopaedic Foot and Ankle Surgeon, Aintree University Hospitals NHS Foundation Trust, University Hospital Aintree, Liverpool, Merseyside, United Kingdom

SELENE G. PAREKH, MD, MBA
Associate Professor, Department of Orthopaedic Surgery, North Carolina Orthopaedic Clinic; and Adjunct Faculty, Fuqua School of Business, Duke University, Durham, North Carolina

CHRISTOPHER J. PEARCE, FRCS (Tr&Orth), MFSEM (UK)
Consultant Orthopaedic Surgeon, Department of Orthopaedics, Jurong Healthcare (Alexandra Hospital), Singapore

TERRY S. SAXBY, MBBS, FRACS (Orth)
Consultant Orthopaedic Surgeon, Brisbane Foot and Ankle Centre, Brisbane Private Hospital, Brisbane, Australia

REINHARD SCHUH, MD
Department of Orthopaedics, Vienna General Hospital, Medical University of Vienna, Vienna, Austria

JAMES SFERRA, MD
Associate Professor, Foot and Ankle Center, Orthopaedic and Rheumatologic Institute, Cleveland Clinic Main Campus, Cleveland, Ohio

RAHEEL SHARIFF, MRCS
Speciality Registrar in Trauma and Orthopaedic Surgery, Mersey Deanery Rotation, St Helens and Knowsley Teaching Hospitals NHS Trust, Prescot, Merseyside, United Kingdom

MATTHEW C. SOLAN, FRCS Tr&Orth
London Foot and Ankle Centre, Hospital of St John and St Elizabeth, London, United Kingdom

HANS JOERG TRNKA, MD
Professor, Foot and Ankle Center, Vienna, Austria

LOWELL SCOTT WEIL SR, DPM
Director, Weil Foot & Ankle Institute, Des Plaines, Illinois

LOWELL WEIL JR, DPM
Research and Fellowship Director, Weil Foot & Ankle Institute, Des Plaines, Illinois

Contents

FORTHCOMING ISSUES

March 2012

Management of the Varus Foot, Ankle, and Tendon
Alastair Younger, MD, *Guest Editor*

June 2012

Adult Flatfoot
Steven M. Raikin, MD, *Guest Editor*

September 2012

Foot & Ankle Innovation in Latin America
Cristian Ortiz, MD, and
Emilio Wagner, MD, *Guest Editors*

December 2012

Total Ankle Replacement
Steven L. Haddad, MD, *Guest Editor*

RECENT ISSUES

September 2011

Tendon Transfers in the Foot and Ankle
Christopher P. Chiodo, MD, and
Eric M. Bluman, MD, PhD, *Guest Editors*

June 2011

Nerve Problems of the Lower Extremity
John S. Gould, MD, *Guest Editor*

March 2011

Current and NewTechniques for Primary and Revision Arthrodesis
Beat Hintermann, MD, *Guest Editor*

Preface

The Lesser Toes

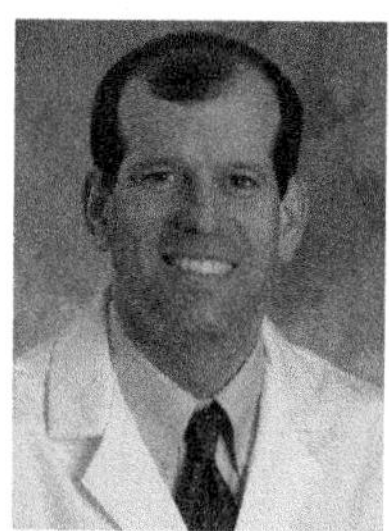

John T. Campbell, MD
Guest Editor

The lesser toes contribute to normal function of the forefoot and to propulsive gait. Disorders of these toes can be difficult for the patient and surgeon alike. Patients suffer pain, dysfunction, and difficulty with footwear, all hallmarks of lesser toe pathology. Surgeons also find these problems troubling, with seemingly simple surgeries complicated by recurrent pain, deformity, and patient dissatisfaction. This issue of *Foot and Ankle Clinics* explores various conditions, considering etiology, evaluation, nonoperative treatment, and surgical options for the lesser toes. A panel of international authors provides outcomes-based recommendations along with personal experience and practical tips to assist the reader in treating these difficult problems.

A series of authors discuss deformities of the lesser toes, including mallet, hammer, claw, and crossover toes. These articles discuss the relevant anatomy and pathophysiology of each condition followed by appropriate evaluation and treatment algorithms. Surgical topics include joint-sparing and fusion techniques, tendon transfers, and metatarsal osteotomies. The treatment of metatarsalgia is also reviewed, considering both distal and proximal metatarsal osteotomies. Common disorders, such as Freiberg's infraction and the bunionette deformity, are also covered in depth.

Congenital lesser toe problems are uncommon, leading to a paucity of literature and relative inexperience among many surgeons. The contributing authors lead the reader through clinical evaluation and treatment options to properly manage these unusual but troubling conditions while minimizing complications. Failed lesser toe surgeries are also covered, guiding the reader through an experienced approach to this frustrating yet little-discussed problem.

A diverse group of experts have contributed to this issue, which is designed to assist surgeons in the treatment of these problems. We hope that our efforts will

Foot Ankle Clin N Am 16 (2011) xi–xii
doi:10.1016/j.fcl.2011.09.003

assist in the treatment of patients, leading ultimately to diminished pain, improved function, and fewer complications.

John T. Campbell, MD
Institute for Foot and Ankle Reconstruction at Mercy
Mercy Medical Center
301 St Paul Place
Baltimore, MD 21202, USA

E-mail address:
jcampbell@mdmercy.com

Mallet Toe Deformity

Andrew Molloy, FRCS Tr&Orth[a,*], Raheel Shariff, MRCS[b]

KEYWORDS

• Mallet • Toe • Lesser • Deformity • Interphalangeal • Joint

Mallet toe is defined as flexion of the distal phalanx over the middle phalanx due to a contracture at the distal interphalangeal joint (DIPJ) (**Fig. 1**).[1–4] The term was first coined by Lake[5] in the orthopedic literature. A mallet toe apart from a sagittal plane deformity described here may also have medial or lateral deviation of the distal phalanx. There is confusion in the orthopedic literature over the definition of the lesser toe deformities, particularly the common ones of hammer toe, clawtoe, and mallet toe.[6] This confusion was shown in a study among Dutch orthopedic surgeons in which there was a lack of consensus in definition and treatment strategies. Although lesser toe surgery is commonly performed, level I evidence and prospective studies are lacking to help determine which procedure is the most successful in achieving good clinical results.[7] The authors offer a practical approach to the diagnosis and treatment of mallet toes for the practicing surgeon.

ANATOMY

The understanding of the extrinsic and intrinsic muscles of the lesser toes and their relationship to the phalanges is crucial for understanding the deformities in this region. The second to fifth toes have three phalanges, whereas the hallux has two. The distal phalanx is the broadest and shortest of the three phalanges and triangular in shape.[8] It supports the germinal and sterile matrices of the overlying nail.[9] It has an oval base for articulation with the trochlear-shaped middle phalangeal head. The base also has tubercles on each side for the insertion of the collateral ligaments. Its tip is described as cauliflower-shaped with a bilobed appearance, which increases the surface area of the tip for weight bearing during the push-off phase of the stance cycle. The distal phalanx has two ossification centers—a primary center in the shaft appearing by the 12th week and a secondary center at the base (epiphysis) arising by the sixth year.[8,10] These two centers fuse by the 18th year.

The authors have nothing to disclose.
[a] Aintree University Hospitals NHS Foundation Trust, University Hospital Aintree, Liverpool, Merseyside, Longmoor Lane, Liverpool, L9 7AL, UK
[b] Trauma and Orthopaedic Surgery, Mersey Deanery Rotation, St Helens and Knowsley Teaching Hospitals NHS Trust, Prescot, Merseyside, UK
* Corresponding author.
E-mail address: orthoblue@aol.com

Foot Ankle Clin N Am 16 (2011) 537–546
doi:10.1016/j.fcl.2011.08.004
1083-7515/11/$ – see front matter

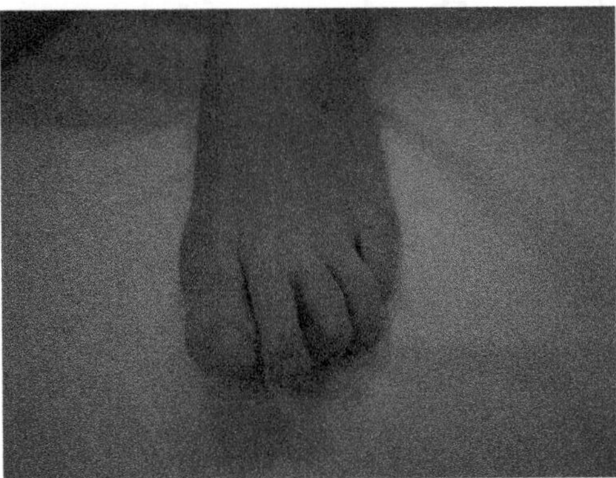

Fig. 1. Mallet third and fourth toes.

The DIPJ is a ginglymus, or a hinge joint. Its normal range of movement is 10° dorsiflexion and 40° plantarflexion.[11] The distal phalanx is controlled by the action of the flexor and extensor tendons, which insert into it (extrinsics) and to a certain extent indirectly by the interossei and lumbricals through their attachment to the extensor hood (**Fig. 2**).[1]

The extensor apparatus to the lesser toes has been well described by Sarrafian and colleagues.[12,13] It consists of the extensor digitorum longus tendon, which divides into three slips at the level of proximal phalanx. The middle slip inserts into the base of the middle phalanx and the two other slips (dorsomedial and dorsolateral) converge and attach at the base of the distal phalanx and act as its principal extensor. The dorsomedial slip is joined by the lumbrical, and the dorsolateral slip is joined by extensor brevis tendon, except for the little toe, which usually does not have a slip from the extensor brevis tendon.[9]. The tendon is encased in a fibroaponeurotic sling

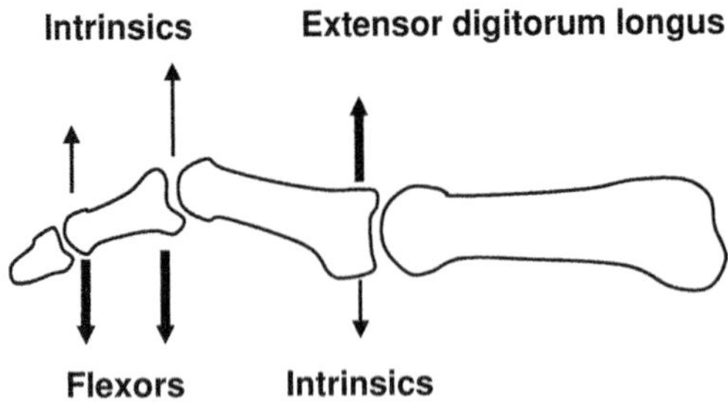

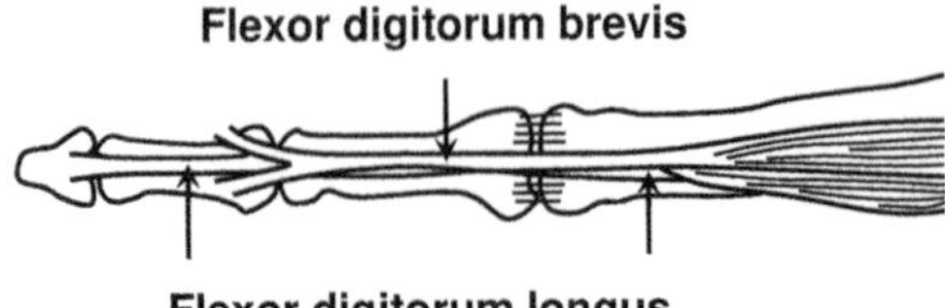

Fig. 2. Muscle actions across the toe and flexor tendon anatomy.

at the level of the metatarsophalangeal joint and extending to the proximal interphalangeal joint level. This "extensor sling" helps keep the tendon in a central position. The tendon is not attached to the proximal phalanx dorsally but via the sling attaches to its plantar surface, thereby acting to dorsiflex the proximal phalanx. It acts to extend the proximal interphalangeal joint only when the proximal phalanx is flexed or in a neutral position. However, when the proximal phalanx is extended, the extensor action of the long extensor tendon is negated on the proximal interphalangeal joint.[4] The "extensor wing," which forms the distal portion of the dorsal extensor complex is a triangular hood that is found on either side of the toe. It has oblique fibers, dorsally being attached to the extensor digitorum longus tendon and its proximal border merging into the extensor sling. The lumbricals form the oblique border of this hood.[12]

The antagonist of the extensor pull on the distal phalanx is by the action of the flexor digitorum longus, the principal extrinsic flexor to the DIPJ. This muscle passes through a tunnel created by two slips of the flexor digitorum brevis at the proximal interphalangeal joint level before inserting into the base of the distal phalanx. The flexor digitorum brevis inserts into the base of the middle phalanx. These two muscles flex the distal and proximal interphalangeal joints, respectively. The flexor tendon is a distinct structure at the level of the distal phalangeal joint.[14]

Apart from the extrinsics, the distal phalanx is also indirectly controlled at the DIPJ by the action of the weaker intrinsic muscles—the lumbricals and the interossei. The interosseous tendons are located dorsal to the transverse metatarsal ligament, and the lumbricals are plantar to it. With respect to the axis of metatarsophalangeal joint motion, both these tendons are plantarward and aid in plantarflexion. These tendons insert into the extensor hood and are dorsal to the axis of motion of the proximal interphalangeal and DIPJs, thereby acting as weak extensors of the distal phalanx.[4,12] The action of the lumbricals is principally to stabilize the proximal phalanx in a plantarward direction. The lumbricals also stabilize the middle phalanx on the proximal phalanx in conjunction with the extensor mechanism. Because the lumbricals originate on the flexor digitorum longus, an excessive pull of the flexor digitorum longus creates increased tension in the lumbricals, further potentiating their action on the middle and proximal phalanx.[15] When external factors such as footwear, muscle imbalance, or idiopathic causes contribute, the long flexors will always overpower the weaker intrinsic muscles, leading to a mallet deformity.[2]

PATHOPHYSIOLOGY/CAUSES

Deformities of the toes are among the most common pathologies affecting the foot and ankle, with incidence reported to range between 2% and 20%.[16–18] The incidence of mallet toe deformity, however, is not as common, accounting for only 5% of lesser toe deformities.[9] Mallet toe deformity occurs at a 1 to 9 ratio compared with hammer toe deformity, as quoted by Coughlin.[19] The deformity has variably been reported to occur in a single toe,[20] although Coughlin[19] and Mann[21] found multiple toe involvement. Coughlin[19] in a series of 60 patients found 11 (18%) had between two to all five toes involved. However, it has been thought that the deformity occurs most frequently in the second or third toe,[21,22] a relatively equal frequency of involvement of the second, third, and fourth toes is usually seen.[19]

The exact cause of mallet toe is unknown.[4,11,14,22] Various causes have been implicated, with the most common being an increased length of the affected toe compared with the adjacent toes.[1–4,19] In 73% of Coughlin's series of 86 toes, the involved toe was found to be longer than the adjacent toes.

The prolonged use of constricting high-heeled foot wear[1,11,23] has also been considered as an important causative factor, acquired mallet toe deformities predominantly found in shoe-wearing Western societies.[1] Up to 84% of affected patients are women, and in Coughlin's series[1–4,19] this factor was found to be highly significant, further strengthening the case for fashionable footwear being implicated A toe longer than the adjacent digits, when constrained in a shoe with a narrow toe box, tends to cause flexion at the DIPJ. With prolonged use, flexion contracture of the flexor digitorum longus may develop, leading to a mallet toe.[2,24] Such deformities, including hammer toes and clawtoes, are usually carried from adulthood into old age but progressively become more severe as degenerative changes set in. Secondary recruitment of toe flexors for propulsion; loss of elasticity of soft tissues, ligaments, and fascia; and attrition of tendons are some of the changes that may exacerbate the changes in old age.[23,25]

Trauma has also been reported as a cause of mallet toe.[11,26–28] Hyperflexion injury of the toe by accidently stubbing it might cause an avulsion of the extensor tendon insertion from the base of the distal phalanx, producing the deformity by unopposed flexor tendon pull.

Inflammatory arthritides have also been proposed as contributing to this deformity, particularly rheumatoid arthritis and psoriatic arthritis.[1,11,14,21] Joint destruction, posttraumatic synovitis, and repeated microtrauma may lead to muscle imbalance and attritional rupture of the extensor mechanism and predispose to the deformity. Deformities secondary to gout and osteoarthritis can also lead to muscle imbalance.[15] Contractures of the deep flexor muscles in the posterior compartment associated with cerebral vascular accident, compartment syndrome, or crush injury may also contribute to the development of the deformity.[15,23] Although usually a sagittal plane deformity, an irregularly shaped middle phalanx (delta phalanx) may lead to medial or lateral deviation of the distal phalanx and also predispose to a mallet toe.[3]

However, in the absence of a bony deformity, a basic imbalance between the flexor and extensor pull can commonly occur in neuromuscular conditions such as cerebral palsy, myelodysplasia, poliomyelitis, Friedreich ataxia, Charcot-Marie-Tooth disease, and multiple sclerosis.[9,11,21] It is therefore prudent to consider such diagnoses when faced with multiple deformities.

Surgery for hammer toe deformity or procedures that aim to shorten the first ray may produce an iatrogenic mallet toe deformity.[4,11] Iatrogenic shortening of the first ray may lead to relative elongation of the second ray, leading to the mallet deformity.

SYMPTOMS

Pain and deformity are the main symptoms of mallet toe. Some patients also seek medical attention for cosmetic purposes.

With the patient weight-bearing, the distal phalanx is often flexed up to 90° at the DIPJ, and pressure at the tip of the distal phalanx causes corns and callosities. Also, the pain in mallet toe deformity occurs at the dorsum of the DIPJ. This pain is because of chronic deformity or inflammatory or idiopathic synovitis of the joint leading to osteophyte formation and pressure symptoms. Repeated microtrauma to the nail bed may also cause nail deformities.[9]

CONSERVATIVE MANAGEMENT

Treatment of mallet toe deformity consists of first assessing the patient for contributing factors such as footwear, presence of neuromuscular disease, and neurovascular sufficiency. Upon examination, it is crucial to assess if the deformity is flexible or fixed. The presence of callosities over the tip of the toe or the dorsum of the DIPJ should also be noted. Conservative means are used before surgical correction is contemplated, particularly in patients with diabetes or peripheral vascular disease. The presence of pressure areas leading to skin breakdown and ulceration should be carefully looked for and prevented. Ulcers, particularly in persons who have diabetes, are the clinical pathway that leads to amputation in 84% of cases.[29]

The deformity is assessed to see if it is flexible or fixed. This assessment should be done with patients standing and sitting. A flexible deformity may cause a flexion deformity of up to 90° at the DIPJ while standing. Upon sitting, with the ankle plantar flexed, the flexible deformity might not be noticeble.[30] In flexible deformities, regular passive stretching of the flexor tendons helps to maintain position and delay further flexion contractures at the DIPJ. Most flexible deformities are managed conservatively, with treatment progressing to surgical options if conservative treatment fails.

Footwear modification is the principal management strategy used, and patients are encouraged to use shoes with wide toe boxes and wider low heels and soft insoles.[1–4,9,14] Callosities or corns are an area of hyperkeratosis that occurs because of intrinsic or extrinsic pressure that develops at the tip of the toe or dorsum of the DIPJ.[31,32] Initial management includes palliative procedures such as removal or trimming of the thickened areas In patients with severe symptoms, the addition of a foam toe crest under the flexor crease of the toe may also be used with good results.[9] Padding may be used for the lesion with various commercially available options including lamb's wool, tube gauze, toe caps, metatarsal bars, foam corn pads, and silicone gel pads.[3] Padding helps to alleviate pain and also prevents pressure symptoms over the skin.

In the acute traumatic mallet toe deformity, nonoperative management can be attempted in the form of extension-splinting the DIPJ for 6 to 10 weeks. However, compared with mallet finger deformities for which conservative means are shown to be effective in 83% of cases, mallet toe deformities do not fare well without surgical fixation.[27]

OPERATIVE TREATMENT

There are two studies in the literature that highlight variations in descriptions of lesser toe deformities.[30,33] However, variation is less with regard to the definition of mallet toes. Barakat and colleagues[30] demonstrated 100% consensus in definition of mallet toe among attending surgeons but only 91% consensus among residents. However, the study by Schrier and colleagues[33] demonstrated that only 70% of respondents were in complete accordance with the definition given by Coughlin and Mann.[34]

This variation is also reflected in the number of procedures described for the correction of this deformity: flexor tenotomy, condylectomy/hemiphalangectomy, resection arthroplasty/fusion, and distal phalanx amputation. Schrier and colleagues[33] demonstrated that these techniques were used to varying degrees by Dutch surgeons. In their study, 58% performed a flexor tenotomy in a flexible deformity, 30% would perform a DIPJ resection arthroplasty, and 58% a DIPJ arthrodesis in a rigid deformity. Three percent would consider an amputation of the distal phalanx in severe cases.

Following is the authors' review of surgical techniques and clinical outcomes and their impressions of each of these techniques.

Flexor Tenotomy

Flexor tenotomy is a frequently discussed and widely used technique. However there is little evidence in the literature to support its use. The majority of reports refer to its usage in curly toes or clawtoes or in conjunction with bony procedures. The only significant series results were published by Kearney and colleagues.[29] Their study

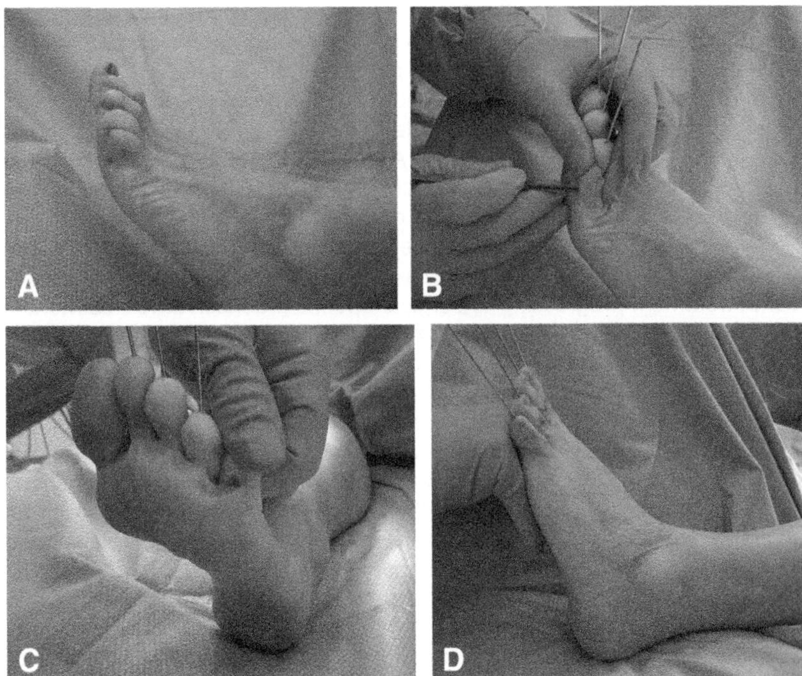

Fig. 3. Operative technique for flexor tenotomy. *(A)* Hammer second to fourth toes with mallet deformity to fourth and fifth toe. *(B)* Incision for flexor tenotomy. *(C)* Post tenotomy. *(D)* Simulated weight bearing after Kirschner wire stabilization.

reported on the use of flexor tenotomy in treatment of ulcers in patients with diabetes mellitus and peripheral neuropathy. There were 58 procedures reported retrospectively with patients being excluded if any additional procedures were performed. Thirty-six percent of their patients had peripheral vascular disease. A total of 98.3% of the procedures healed, with 1 patient (1.7%) requiring amputation because of preexisting osteomyelitis. A total of 5.2% of patients developed postoperative infections. There was recurrence of ulceration in 12.1% of toes.

The authors only use this technique as an isolated procedure if there is a flexible deformity of less than 45°. One needs to assess for dorsal osteophytes at the DIPJ because these prevent correction of the deformity. If there is any doubt, or if correction can only be achieved under tension, then an adjunctive bony procedure is also performed.

Technique

The procedure can be performed under a local anaesthetic block with a general anaesthetic being reserved for cases in which multiple other procedures are being performed (**Fig. 3**). If flexor tenotomy is the sole procedure, a tourniquet is not necessary. A transverse incision is performed on the plantar aspect at the level of the distal flexor crease. Care needs to be taken to remain on the plantar surface so as not to damage the neurovascular bundles. The long flexor is transected so that the blade comes to rest against bone. Gentle pressure is applied to the toe until the DIPJ is in neutral extension. This action will leave a diamond-shaped defect in the skin. The defect is not closed because skin contracture, in the authors' opinion, is part of the deforming process. If the defect is small, the toe can simply be taped into extension. However, if there is a larger skin defect, a Kirschner wire is used to support the correction for 3 to 4 weeks. Patients are advised to mobilize in a stiff-soled sandal until the skin defect has epithelialized.

Hemiphalangectomy/Condylectomy

The hemiphalangectomy/condylectomy technique has been most commonly described for the treatment of hammer toe, with good results being reported. Although the technique has been described for mallet toe,[9] there are no series of published results for mallet toe correction alone. The authors believe that the fibrous union is not as stable, takes longer to mature, and is not as predictable as a DIPJ arthrodesis. This technique is therefore not advocated by the authors.

Technique

The hemiphalangectomy/condylectomy technique, as described by Murphy[9] involves an elliptical incision over the DIPJ, with a smaller ellipse being excised from the dorsal hood. The extensor hood is then elevated off the middle phalanx to enable later repair. The collateral ligaments are divided, and the head of the middle phalanx is delivered into the incision. Sufficient bone is then resected to enable tension-free alignment in a neutral position. An adjunctive flexor tenotomy may then be performed if necessary. Correction can be maintained by repair of the extensor hood and a dorsal dermodesis. A retrograde Kirschner wire may also be used for stabilization.

DIPJ Resection Arthroplasty/Arthrodesis

The first report of a toe interphalangeal joint fusion was by Soule[35] in 1910. The definitive article on treatment of mallet toe deformity using this technique was by Coughlin.[19] Coughlin reported on a series of 72 toes that underwent resection arthroplasty in which the middle phalanx at the supracondylar region and the articular surface of the distal phalanx were resected to promote bony fusion. A flexor tenotomy was also performed in the most severe cases. Successful arthrodesis was achieved in 72% of toes, with a fibrous union (resection arthroplasty) being present in the remaining 28%. Overall patient satisfaction was 86%. However, the satisfaction rate was lower, 75%, if a fibrous union was present. At a mean of 55 months, acceptable alignment was present in 96% of cases in which a flexor tenotomy was not necessary (the milder cases) and in 90% in which a flexor tenotomy was deemed necessary because of the severity of the deformity. Pain was relieved in 97% of cases. Minor complications occurred in 14% of toes. These complications included numbness, instability of the DIPJ, and deviation of the digit (including development of a hammer toe and hyperextension at the DIPJ). This technique remains the most commonly performed procedure by the authors.

Technique

The authors use the technique described by Coughlin[19] (**Fig. 4**). A digital block and a toe tourniquet are used except where general anesthesia is thought to be preferable because of multiple other procedures being performed.

An elliptical incision centered over the dorsal surface of the DIPJ is used. The underlying extensor tendon and capsule are also elliptically excised and the collateral ligaments released. It is prudent to keep the blade parallel to the phalanges to prevent neurovascular damage. One should also not stray too distally so as to prevent damage to the nail matrix. The head of the middle phalanx is delivered into the incision

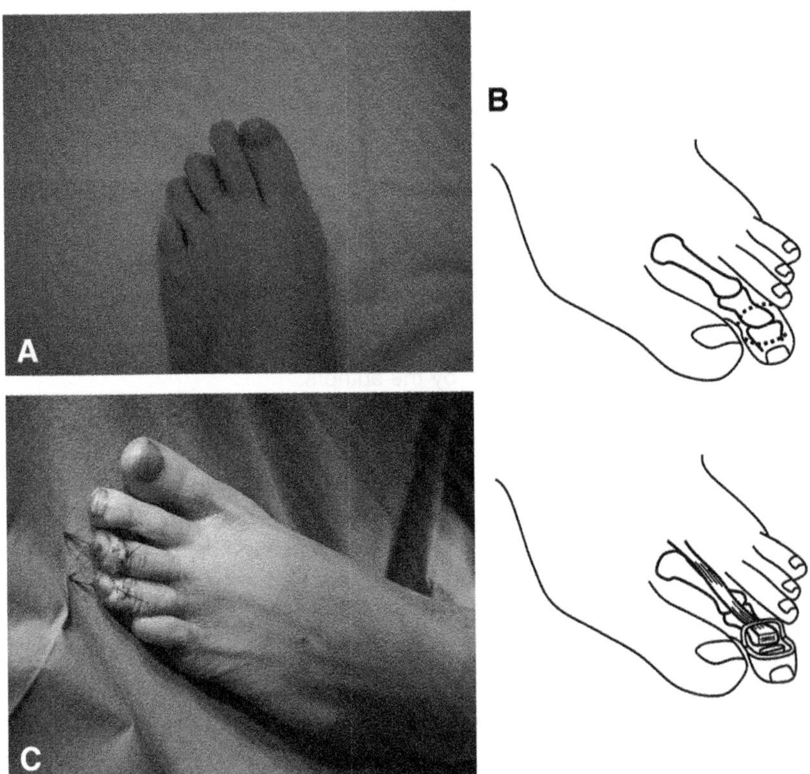

Fig. 4. Operative technique for resection arthroplasty/arthrodesis. (*A*) Mallet third and fourth toes. (*B*) Incision and bony resection. (*C*) Post Kirschner wire stabilization.

and is resected in the supracondylar region with bone cutters. Care needs to be taken to make the plane of resection perpendicular to the axis of the toe. The corresponding articular surface of the distal phalanx is also resected in the same plane. In severe cases of deformity in which bony decompression has not achieved a toe that can be straightened without tension, a flexor tenotomy is also performed under direct vision. If a tension-free correction is still difficult to achieve, further bone should be resected form the middle phalanx. A Kirschner wire is used to maintain correction. The wire is driven in an antegrade fashion from the base of the distal phalanx out through the tip of the toe, then back retrograde across the DIPJ so as to ensure that the wire is exactly centered. The authors find that stability is better if the tip of the wire reaches just distal to the base of the middle phalanx. That stability is better is especially true in patients with osteopenia or osteoporosis. Sutures are removed at 2 weeks and the wire at 4 weeks. Taping can be used for up to a further 6 weeks if bony union has not been achieved by the 4-week stage.

Distal Phalangectomy

There is one modern series reporting on the outcome of amputation by Raja and colleagues.[36] This report is a retrospective review of 26 patients (39 toes) with a mean age of 63 years. All patients had satisfactory pain relief. A total of 97% patients were wholly satisfied, with 3% (1 patient) being satisfied with minor reservations. The complication rate was 7.5%, which included minor wound infection and asymptomatic nail growth from a nail matrix remnant.

This is a technique used sparingly by the authors. It is usually reserved for the most elderly patients who have requested amputation or those with severe comorbidities that would almost certainly lead to complications from other techniques (eg. severe arteriopathy or fulminant osteomyelitis).

Technique

This technique is normally performed under local anaesthesia with a toe tourniquet. Careful hemostasis is essential for preventing painful swelling or even wound breakdown. A long plantar flap is preferably used so as to keep the incision away from the tip of the stump where it may cause painful symptoms. The DIPJ is disarticulated, and the flap is used to cover the stump. Nonabsorbable sutures are removed at 2 weeks.

SUMMARY

Mallet toe is one of the most common deformities encountered by orthopedic surgeons. Care needs to be taken to ascertain whether it is a primary condition or secondary to a systemic disease, especially if multiple deformities are present. There are numerous operative strategies available, but each has its specific indications. If the indications are followed, highly successful outcomes may be achieved.

REFERENCES

1. Coughlin MJ. Mallet toes, hammer toes, claw toes, and corns. Causes and treatment of lesser-toe deformities. Postgrad Med 1984;75(5):191–8.
2. Coughlin MJ. Lesser toe deformities. Orthopedics 1987;10(1):63–75.
3. Coughlin MJ. Lesser toe abnormalities. J Bone Joint Surg Am 2002;84:1446–69.
4. Coughlin MJ. Lesser toe abnormalities. In: Coughlin MJ, Mann RA, editors. Surgery of the foot and ankle. 8th edition. Philadelphia: Mosby Elsevier; 2007. p. 364.
5. Lake N. Hallux rigidus, hallux flexus and hammertoes. In: The foot. 2nd edition. Baltimore (MD): Williams & Wilkins; 1939. p. 206.
6. Schrier JC, Louwerens JW, Verheyen CC. Opinions on lesser toe deformities among Dutch orthopaedic departments. Foot Ankle Int 2007;28(12):1265–70.
7. Harmonson JK, Harkless LB. Operative procedures for the correction of hammertoe, claw toe, and mallet toe: a literature review. Clin Podiatr Med Surg 1996 Apr; 13(2):211–20.
8. Chan R. Anatomy of the digits. Clin Podiatr Med Surg 1986;3(1):3–9.
9. Murphy GA. Mallet toe deformity. Foot Ankle Clin 1998;3:279.
10. Standring S, editor. Gray's anatomy. The anatomical basis of clinical practice. 39th edition. Philadelphia: Elsevier; 2005. p. 1514.
11. Helal B, Rowley DI, Cracchiolo A III et al, editors. Surgery of disorders of the foot and ankle. London: Martin Dunitz Ltd; 1996. p. 336.
12. Sarrafian SK, Toprizian WK. Anatomy and physiology of the extensor apparatus of the toes. J Bone Joint Surg Am 1969;51A:669–79.
13. Sarrafian SK. Anatomy of the foot and ankle. Philadelphia: JB Lippincott; 1983.
14. Mizel M. Anatomy and pathophysiology of the lesser toes. In: Gould JS, editor, Operative foot surgery. Philadelphia: WB Saunders; 1993, p. 84–5.
15. Morris JL. Biomechanical implications of hammertoe deformities. Clin Podiatr Med Surg 1986;3(2):339–46.
16. Cooper PS. Disorders and deformities of the lesser toes. In: Myerson MS, editor, Foot and ankle disorders. Philadelphia; WB Saunders; 2000. p. 308–58.

17. Hewitt D, Stewart A, Webb J. The prevalence of foot defects amongst wartime recruits. Br Med J 1953;2:745–9.
18. Lamberinudi C. The feet of the industrial worker. Lancet 1938;2:1480–4.
19. Coughlin MJ. Operative treatment of the mallet toe deformity, Foot Ankle Int 1995; 16(3):109-16.
20. Brahm M. The small toes. In: Disorders of the foot and ankle. Philadelphia: WB Saunders; 1991. p. 1187.
21. Mann RA, Coughlin MJ. Lesser toe deformities. Instr Course Lect 1987;36:137–59.
22. Ishikawa S, Murphy GA. Lesser toe abnormalities. In: Canale ST, Beaty JH, editors, Campbells operative orthopaedics. 11th edition. Philadelphia: Mosby Elsevier; 2008. p. 4625.
23. Femino JE, Mueller K. Complications of lesser toe surgery. Clin Orthop Relat Res 2001;391:72–88.
24. Coughlin MJ. Lesser toe abnormalities. In: Chapman MW, editor. Operative orthopaedics. Philadelphia: Lippincott; 1988. p 1765–76.
25. Caselli MA, George DH. Foot deformities: biomechanical and pathomechanical changes associated with aging, Part I. Clin Podiatr Med Surg 2003;20(3):487–509.
26. Hennessey MS, Saxby TS. Traumatic 'mallet toe' of the hallux: a case report. Foot Ankle Int 2001;22(12):977–8.
27. Lancaster SC. Acute mallet toe. Clin J Sports Med 2008;18:298–9.
28. Nakamura S. Temporary Kirschner wire fixation for a mallet toe of the hallux. J Orthop Sci 2007;12(2):190–2.
29. Kearney TP. Safety and efficacy of flexor tenotomy for ulcers in persons with DM. Diabetes Res Clin Pract 2010;89:224–6.
30. Barakat MJ, Gargan MF. Deformities of the lesser toes—how should we describe them? Foot 2006;16(1):16–8.
31. Coughlin MJ, Kennedy MP. Operative repair of fourth and fifth toe corns. Foot Ankle Int 2003;24(2):147–57.
32. Brahms M. Common foot problems. J Bone Joint Surg Am 1967;49A:1653–64.
33. Schrier JC, Verheyen CC, Louwerens JW. Definitions of hammer toe and claw toe: an evaluation of literature. J Am Podiatr Med Assoc 2009;99(3):194–7.
34. Coughlin MJ, Mann R, editors. Surgery of the foot and ankle. St Louis (MO): Mosby; 1999. p. 320–72.
35. Soule R. Operation for the treatment of hammer toe and claw toe. J Bone Joint Surg Am 1938;20(3):608–9.
36. Raja S, Barrie JL, Henderson AA. Distal phalangectomy for mallet toe. Foot and Ankle Surgery 2003;9(4):215–6.

Hammertoes and Clawtoes: Proximal Interphalangeal Joint Correction

J. Kent Ellington, MD, MS[a,b,c,*]

KEYWORDS

• Hammertoe • Clawtoe • PIP • Correction

Lesser toe deformities are a common complaint. Lesser toe pathology can be erroneously considered a minor problem, because pain and deformity can have a significant impact on a patient's quality of life. Hammertoes and clawtoes are the most common deformity; surgical management of these deformities is among the most common procedures performed on the forefoot.[1]

The etiology of hammertoes and clawtoes include intrinsic muscle imbalance, neuromuscular conditions including diabetes and lumbar disc disease, overcrowding in the shoe's toebox, hallux valgus, excessively long metatarsals, posttraumatic sequela, congenital deformity, and inflammatory arthropathies. Regardless of the cause, there are common anatomic similarities which guide treatment options, both nonoperative and operative.

PATHOLOGIC ANATOMY OF HAMMERTOES AND CLAWTOES

The lesser toes are important for pressure distribution and balance of the foot. Deformities lead to pain, callous formation, transfer lesions, and compensatory gait changes. Initially, the deformity is flexible, but as it progresses, it may become more rigid. A basic understanding of the anatomy of the lesser toes is important to better appreciate the pathologic changes that occur with hammertoes and clawtoes.

For the purpose of this discussion, hammertoes are defined as flexion of the proximal interphalangeal (PIP) joint with or without distal interphalangeal (DIP) joint

---

Disclosure: The author did not receive any direct payments, outside funding, or grants in support of research or for the preparation of this manuscript. However, some of the implants discussed in the article are produced by Wright Medical Inc., which provides research funding to the author's institution.

[a] Foot and Ankle Institute, OrthoCarolina, 2001 Vail Ave, Charlotte, NC 28207, USA
[b] University of North Carolina—Charlotte, Charlotte, NC 28223, USA
[c] Department of Orthopaedic Surgery, Carolinas Medical Center, 1000 Blythe Boulevard, Charlotte, NC 28203, USA
* Corresponding author. Foot and Ankle Institute, OrthoCarolina, 2001 Vail Ave, Charlotte, NC 28207.
E-mail address: kentellington@yahoo.com

Foot Ankle Clin N Am 16 (2011) 547–558
doi:10.1016/j.fcl.2011.08.010
1083-7515/11/$ – see front matter

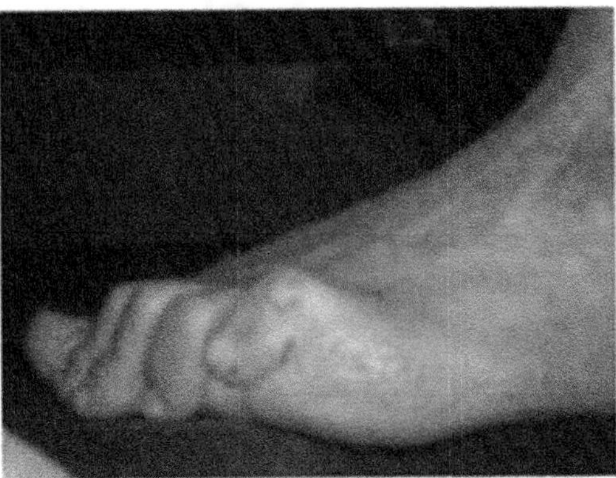

Fig. 1. Hammertoes. Note the flexion of the PIP joints.

involvement (**Fig. 1**). Clawtoes are defined as extension of the metatarsophalangeal (MP) joint with flexion of the PIP and DIP joints (**Fig. 2**). In addition, clawtoes are frequently associated with neuromuscular conditions (see **Fig. 2**) , usually involving multiple lesser toes bilaterally; in contrast, hammertoes can occur in isolation, with the second toe most commonly affected.[2]

Hammertoe and clawtoe deformities occur with simultaneous contracture of the long flexors and extensors of the toe, with imbalance and overpowering of the intrinsic muscles.[3] The extensor digitorum longus tendon divides into 3 slips over the proximal phalanx. The middle slips inserts onto the base of the middle phalanx and the 2 lateral slips pass lateral and converge to form the terminal tendon inserting on the base of the distal phalanx (**Fig. 3**).[4,5]

The flexor digitorum longus (FDL) tendon inserts onto the distal phalanx, flexing the DIP. The flexor digitorum brevis tendon inserts onto the middle phalanx, flexing the PIP joint. There is no direct flexor insertion on the proximal phalanx; thus, with the MP joint in the extended position, there are no antagonists, resulting in flexion in the PIP and DIP.

The transverse metatarsal ligament divides the intrinsic musculature, with the interossei dorsal to the ligament and the lumbricals plantar. However, both muscles are plantar to the MP joint axis, resulting in flexion of the MP joint; the intrinsics pass dorsal to the PIP and DIP joint axis, extending these joints.

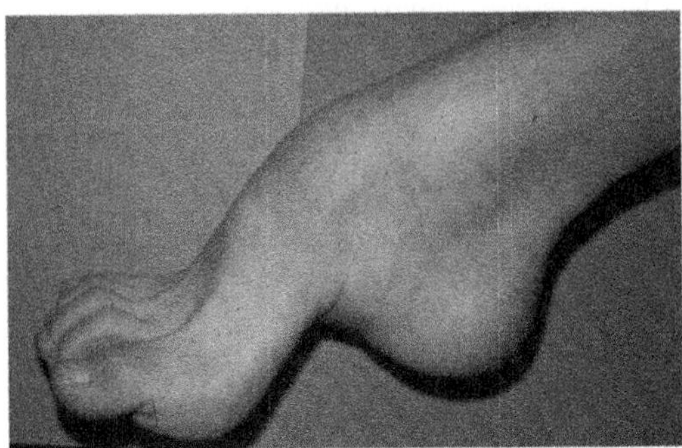

Fig. 2. Clawtoes. Note the typical cavus associated with this condition.

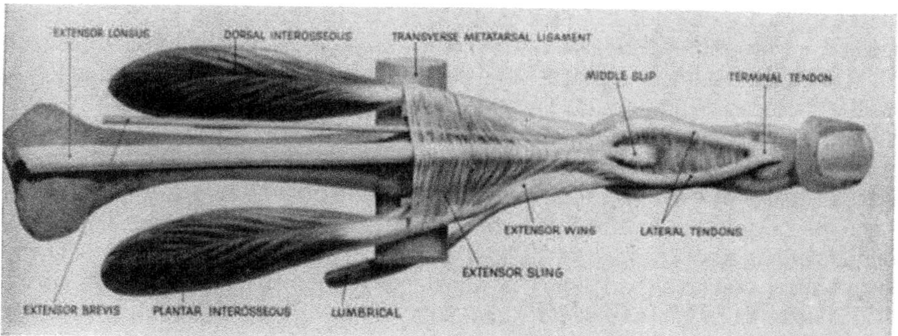

Fig. 3. Lesser toe anatomy. Lateral view of the metatarsal and phalanges. (*From* Mizel MS, Yodlowski ML. Disorders of the lesser metatarsophalangeal joints. J Am Acad Orthop Surg 1995;3: 166-173. © 1995 American Academy of Orthopaedic Surgeons. Reprinted with permission.)

The MP joint is frequently involved in these deformities as well. The MP joint is stabilized by collateral ligaments and the plantar plate, which limit dorsiflexion of the MP joint during gait. The plantar plate inserts distally on the proximal phalanx and proximally onto the plantar fascia. As the deformity progresses, the plantar plate attenuates and leads to subluxation of the proximal phalanx dorsally onto the metatarsal head. This in turn pulls the metatarsal fat pad distally and depresses the metatarsal head plantarly, leading to painful metatarsalgia.

Hammertoes and clawtoes result from an imbalance between the strong extrinsics and weak intrinsics. With the proximal phalanx in the neutral position, the extensor digitorum longus extends the PIP and DIP joints while the FDL flexes the MP joint. However, when the proximal phalanx is extended, the extensor digitorum longus loses its tenodesing effect, which allows the PIP and DIP to flex from the unopposed long flexor. The only counteracting extensors of the IP joints are the lumbricals and interossei, but these are weak and easily overpowered by the stronger extrinsics. Additionally, the intrinsics are off axis owing to the extension of the MP joint. Coupled with attenuation of the passive stabilizers (plantar plate, collateral ligaments, joint capsule), this leads to hyperextension of the proximal phalanx, described by Coughlin and Mann[6] as the key to these deformities. Hyperextension of the proximal phalanx is integral to the evolution of the deformity, substantiated by several reasons. During gait, the ground reactive forces are forcing the proximal phalanx dorsally on the MP joint. Second, the toe extensors are active during 65% of the gait cycle and unopposed during 50%.[7] Third, it helps to explain why these deformities occur in shoe-wearing societies, particularly in patients who wear higher heeled shoes, and with advanced age.[6,8–10]

PHYSICAL EXAMINATION/RADIOGRAPHS

In evaluating the patient, both standing and seated foot examinations are crucial. Visual inspection identifies deformity and malalignment of the lesser toes in the standing position, as many deformities cannot be truly appreciated solely during the seated examination. In addition, the position of the hallux should be evaluated for possible contribution to lesser toe abnormalities. Examination of the skin identifies callosities or ulcerations dorsally over the PIP joint, distally at the tip of the toe, or plantarly under the MP joint. A careful examination of the neurovascular status is important, because neurologic conditions may be the underlying etiology; it is also necessary to ensure adequate tissue perfusion for successful healing. In the seated position, it is possible to determine whether the deformity is rigid or flexible, because this may alter treatment options. A flexible deformity corrects when the ankle is passively placed in the neutral position, whereas a rigid toe deformity does not correct. Last, the stability of the MP joint should be tested with the vertical drawer test. The examiner stabilizes the metatarsal and shucks the phalanx vertically to assess stability of the joint; this is compared with the contralateral foot as a control. Standard weightbearing radiographs of the foot are obtained, including anteroposterior, lateral, and oblique views. Overall forefoot alignment is evaluated, identifying hallux valgus, metatarsus adductus, and the relative lengths of the lesser metatarsals. Flexion deformities of the lesser toes are readily noted, often with a "gun barrel" sign in cases of severe toe flexion.

NONSURGICAL TREATMENT

Nonsurgical treatment is initially attempted in most instances. Patients with hammertoes or clawtoes are encouraged to wear shoes with wide toe boxes to accommodate the deformities and alleviate impingement of the digits. Shoes with high heels are discouraged, because they transfer increased pressure to the afflicted forefoot. Taping or strapping of the affected toes may improve alignment if they are flexible, although these techniques do not provide a permanent solution because the deformity recurs once the tape or strapping device is removed. Padding of painful calluses with felt or silicone gel pads can relieve impingement over bony prominences. Periodic trimming or shaving of painful calluses may also be helpful. Finally, nonsteroidal anti-inflammatory medications may provide analgesia.

PIP CORRECTION

The surgeon must customize the approach to each patient to address the deformity at the involved levels to obtain a successful correction. In some instances, correction through the DIP and MP joints are necessary, which is discussed in other articles. For example, full correction may require addressing the PIP joint as well as concomitant extensor tenotomy and MP joint capsulotomy to achieve a satisfactory outcome.

Correction of the PIP joint itself can be performed with a variety procedures: Soft tissue capsulotomy, tendon release or transfer, proximal phalangeal condylectomy, PIP arthroplasty, PIP arthrodesis, diaphysectomy, silicone implant, amputation, and partial proximal phalangectomy. In addition, numerous fixation techniques have been described. These include the use of pins, wires, screws, bone dowels, bioabsorbable pins, digital implants, and intramedullary implants.[11–21] This review describes different PIP correction procedures with various fixation methods. Tendon transfer techniques are discussed in a separate article.

Correction of the PIP Joint

The 2 most common procedures are PIP resection arthroplasty and PIP arthrodesis. Both have advantages and disadvantages, which the surgeon must consider. Although the author prefers PIP arthrodesis, PIP arthroplasty is advantageous in that it retains some motion. Perhaps in the younger, active, or athletic patient, PIP arthroplasty may be beneficial. However, motion may lead to pain or the chance for recurrent deformity, thus not alleviating the entire problem for the patient. On the other hand, PIP arthrodesis can be in patients with neuropathy or an underlying neurologic disorder, which may increase the risk of recurrent deformity. A PIP arthrodesis may provide a more stable, pain-free construct over time. In addition, the author recommends it for the revision situation as well.

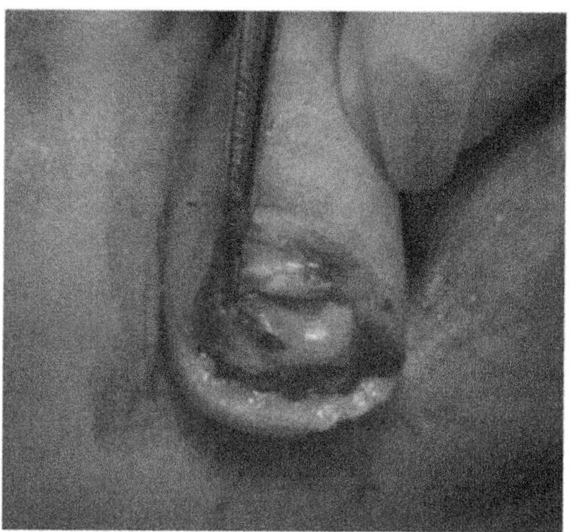

Fig. 4. Release of the collateral ligaments.

Both procedures are performed by making a longitudinal or transverse elliptical incision over the PIP joint. The author prefers a transverse elliptical incision to remove redundant skin after shortening of the toe. The extensor tendon and hood are similarly excised and the collateral ligaments are released (**Fig. 4**). The distal portion of the proximal phalanx is resected with a bone cutter or saw (**Fig. 5**). If an arthrodesis is planned, the middle phalanx is then prepared by removing the cartilage with a small rongeur or curet.

It is important, regardless of technique, to have a parallel PIP joint after bone resection to prevent varus–valgus or flexion–extension deformity. Most commonly, the bone cuts are made transversely; however, other techniques have been described. A sagittal plane chevron and "V" arthrodesis has been reported with

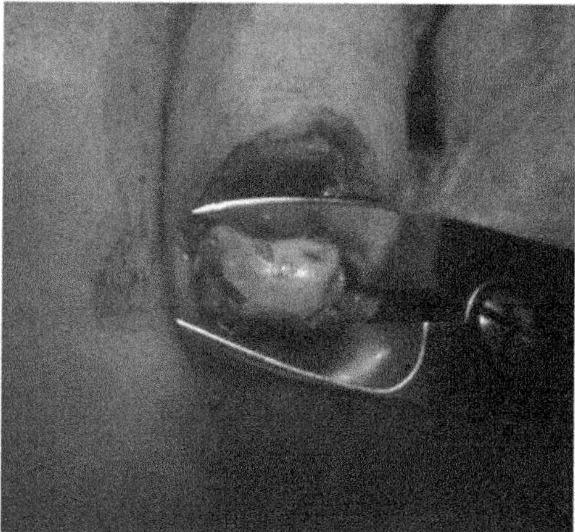

Fig. 5. Resection of the distal end of the proximal phalanx with a bone cutter.

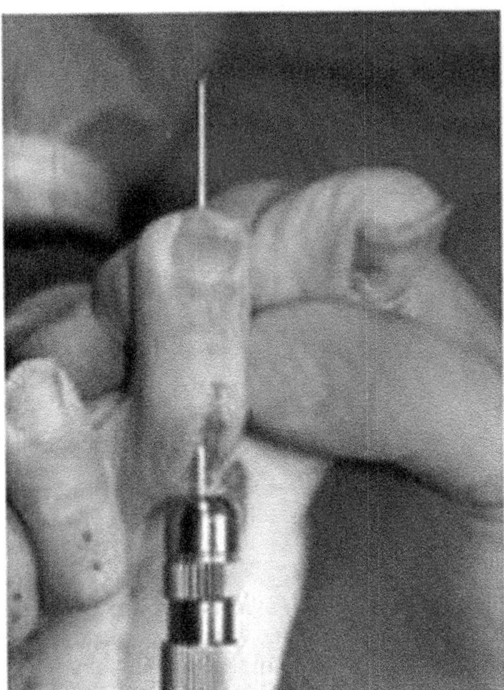

Fig. 6. Passing the K-wire out the tip of the toe initially (anterograde).

favorable results.[21–23] Although this adds to the complexity of the case, the authors state that this technique adds to the stability of the construct and increases bony surface area to promote earlier union.[21] Also, a peg-in-hole technique has been shown to be superior to both transverse cuts and the "V" construct, but this approach is technically more difficult with the increased risk of dorsal cortex fracture.[23–27] Lamm and colleagues[16] evaluated 177 toes and found no difference between the peg-in-hole technique versus the end-to-end method.

After preparation of the PIP joint, a tenotomy of the FDL tendon can easily be performed through the dorsal incision if the surgeon feels the contracted tendon may predispose to recurrent contracture of the toe. A scalpel blade is passed through the PIP joint to transect the FDL tendon, with care taken to avoid penetrating the plantar skin of the toe or straying too medial or lateral potentially jeopardizing the neurovascular bundles. After joint preparation, the PIP joint is stabilized. Historically, a K-wire has been chosen with good results, as described. The K-wire is driven anterograde out the tip of the toe (**Fig. 6**) then retrograde across the PIP joint (**Fig. 7**). There are several disadvantages to using K-wires. The greatest disadvantage is the inconvenience to the patient by having exposed hardware and the risks associated with this (breakage, migration, accidental removal). In addition, K-wires pose an increased risk of infection, possible loss of correction, and the anxiety and potential pain experienced by the patient when the K-wires are removed in the clinic setting. Thus, several alternatives have been developed to address these shortcomings. These include resection arthroplasty or arthrodesis with pins, wires, screws, bone dowels, bioabsorbable pins, intramedullary devices, and digital implants.[12,14–18,20,28]

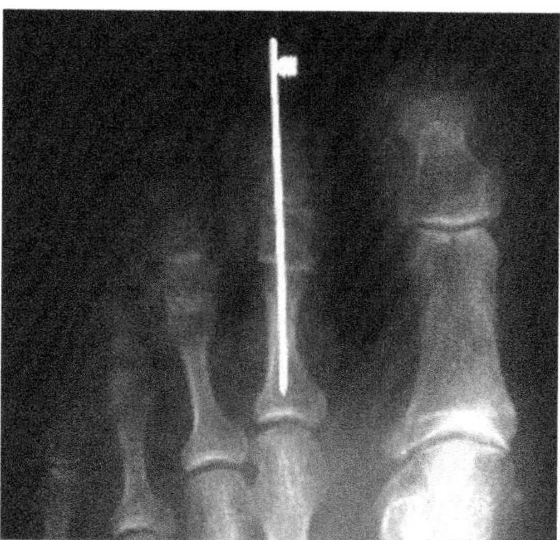

Fig. 7. Hammertoe correction fixed with a K-wire.

Coughlin reported on 118 toes with approximately 5-year follow-up after PIP resection arthroplasty and placement of K-wire for a fixed hammertoe deformity. There was a fibrous union in 19% and radiographic alignment was good in only 79%. However, 92% of the patients reported good pain relief and 86% were satisfied with the clinical alignment of the toe, emphasizing that pain relief and correction of the deformity are more important than a successful fusion.[29] Alvine and Garvin[14] reported on 73 toes using the peg and dowel fusion method with a 97% fusion rate and 87% favorable outcomes.[11] Konkel and associates[14] used an intramedullary absorbable pin in 48 toes. They reported a bony union of 73% and a fibrous union of 19%; patient

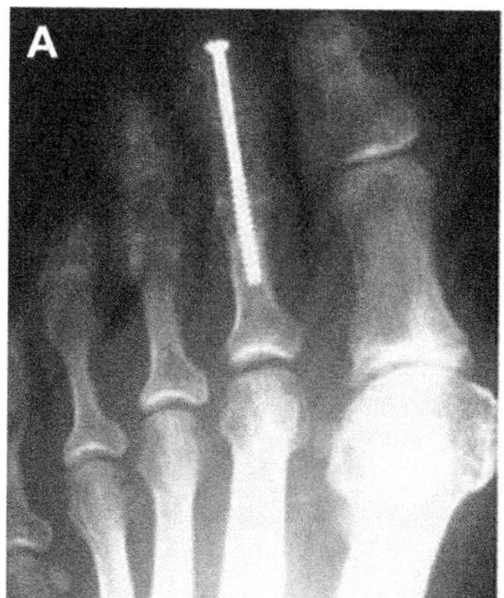

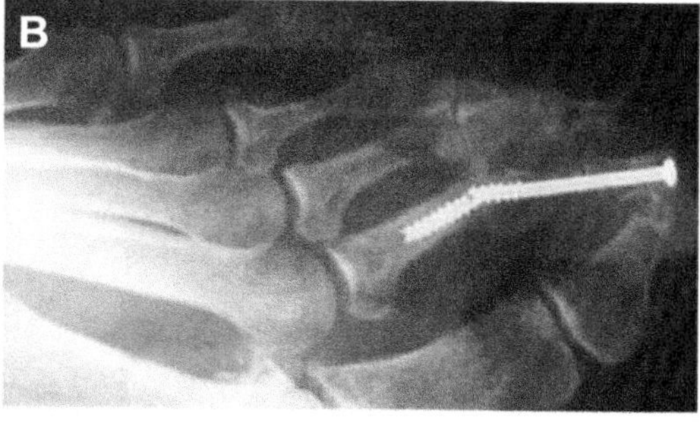

Fig. 8. (*A*) Intramedullary screw placed for hammertoe correction. (*B*) Broken screw. (*From* Caterini R, et al. Arthrodesis of the toe joints with an intramedullary cannulated screw for correction of hammertoe deformity. Foot Ankle Int 2004;25:256–61. Copyright © 2004 by the American Orthopaedic Foot and Ankle Society, Inc.; with permission.)

satisfaction rating was 91%. Importantly, no hyperextension deformity was noted; thus, no painful recurvatum occurred. Floating toe occurred in 19% and angulation was present in 17% of the toes. Pietrzak and co-workers[17] biomechanically compared a threaded/barbed bioabsorbable fixation implant made of a copolymer of 82% poly-L-lactic acid and 18% polyglycolic acid with a 1.57-mm Kirschner wire using the devices to fix 2 synthetic bone blocks together.[17] Constructs were evaluated by applying a cantilever load. No device fractured with testing. These results suggest that the bioabsorbable implant would be a suitable fixation device for the hammer toe procedure. Caterini and colleagues[28] reported on 51 hammertoes fixed with an intramedullary screw. A fusion was noted in 94% and 1 screw had broken (**Fig. 8**). Hardware was removed in 29% of patients; however, they concluded that this method was superior because no infections were observed and a higher union rate was achieved.

Recently, we reported on an intramedullary fusion device in 38 toes.[20] The device was effective in maintaining coronal alignment in 87% of cases and sagittal alignment in 95% (**Fig. 9**). A solid bony union was observed in 61% and the device broke in 8%. In addition, no patient required a second surgery owing to hardware pain, which was

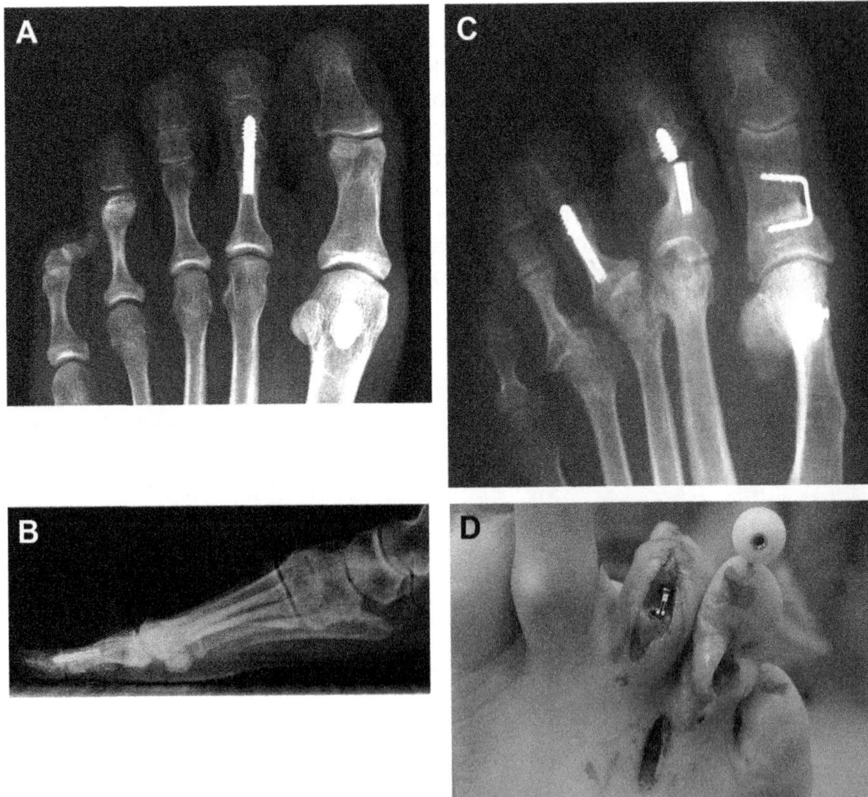

Fig. 9. (*A*) Successful outcome with the 2-piece intramedullary device. (*B*) Lateral radiograph. (*C*) Hardware failure and loss of alignment requiring revision surgery. (*D*) The 2-piece design and engagement of the distal end into the proximal end.

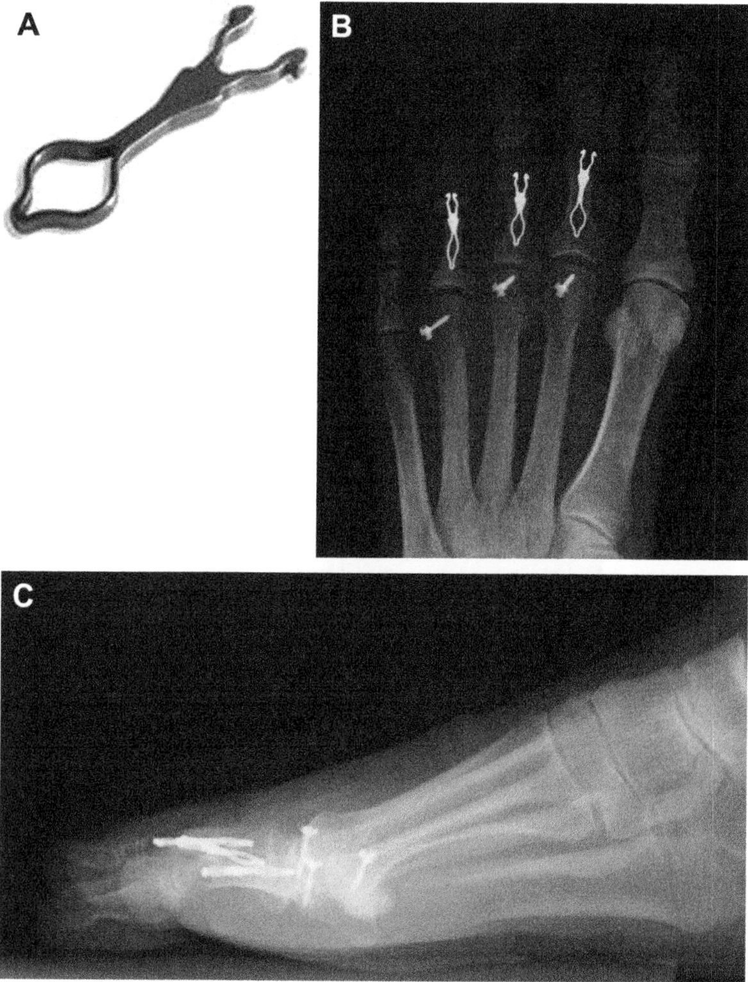

Fig. 10. (*A*) Memory clip device thermally activated upon placement. (*B*) The memory clips with a successful outcome. (*C*) Lateral radiograph.

an advantage of this device. Also, we have experience using 2 other intramedullary devices. One is thermally activated. This implant helps to achieve proper fusion because of the compressive properties made possible by its temperature-activated material, NiTinol alloy. The implant is cooled before surgery, and once implanted, the body heat expands its width and shortens its length. Expansion secures the implant in place, and the shortening pulls the bones tightly together to maintain bony contact. There are no reports of this device; however, our experience has been positive (**Fig. 10**). Its advantage over the previously mentioned intramedullary device is that is a 1-piece implant with 0° and 10° flexion options; no connection is required intraoperatively. Last, we have experience with a newer, 1-piece intramedullary device that also comes in 0° and 10° flexion options and varying sizes. We have used this during the last year in premarket trials with good success as well (**Fig. 11**).

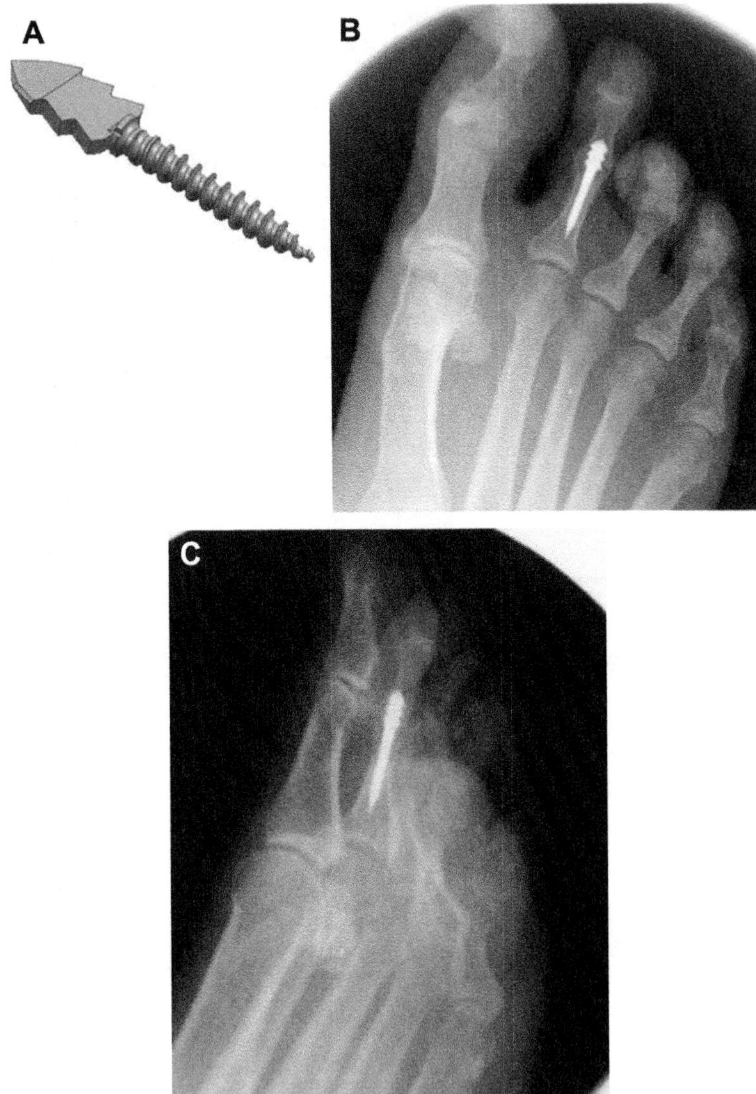

Fig. 11. (*A*) The 1-piece intramedullary device. (*B*) Radiographic image. (*C*) Oblique radiograph.

Complications

Complications of PIP correction is a frustrating problem for both patient and surgeon. These include swelling, numbness, pain, stiffness, hardware problems, malalignment, and even loss of the toe owing to vascular insult. Radiographic results can sometimes be discordant with clinical outcomes, because x-rays may show a well-aligned toe, but patient satisfaction may be poor. If a nonunion is present, revision PIP arthrodesis is the best salvage. Likewise, this is a good option in a malaligned toe. Intramedullarly hardware complications are usually best resolved with revision using a K-wire, whereas failed previous surgery with a K-wire may be best handled with revision using an intramedullary device.

ALTERNATIVE PROCEDURES

There are other options for PIP correction; however, these are often reserved for severe deformities and for revision procedures. These include diaphysectomy,[30,31] partial proximal phalangectomy,[32–34] and amputation as salvage.[35,36] These options have been reported with moderate success and are mentioned mainly for historical interests. However, digital amputation can be an excellent salvage for the patient with multiple previous failed hammertoe corrections, particularly in an elderly or sedentary patient population.

SUMMARY

Hammertoe and clawtoe deformities are common forefoot problems. The deformity exists owing to the underlying pathoanatomy. Hallux valgus, longer metatarsals, and intrinsic imbalance are the most common etiologies. Understanding the cause of the deformity is important to be able to successfully treat the condition, whether nonoperative or with operative intervention. When nonoperative measures fail, PIP correction is best obtained through arthroplasty or arthrodesis.

The key to successful PIP correction is obtaining a well-aligned toe and reducing pain as demonstrated by Coughlin and Mann.[15] When choosing a technique, the author prefers PIP joint arthrodesis because it has several advantages, including a decreased risk of recurrence and a more predictable toe posture. The authors prefers an intramedullary device to avoid the well-known complications of K-wires. The best surgical correction and fixation techniques are still to be determined. Each patient much be evaluated thoroughly and treatment should be tailored to the patient's deformity, comorbidities, expectations and surgeon's experience.

REFERENCES

1. Coughlin M, Dorris J, Polk E. Operative repair of the fixed hammertoe deformity. Foot Ankle Int 2000;21:94–104.
2. Canale ST. Campbell's operative orthopaedics. Philadelphia: Mosby; 2003. p. 4051.
3. Scheck M. Etiology of acquired hammertoe deformity. Clin Ortho Relat Res 1977;123: 63–9.
4. Sarrafian S. Correction of fixed hammertoe deformity with resection of the head of the proximal phalanx and extensor tendon tenodesis. Foot Ankle Int 1995;16:449–51.
5. Saffarian S, Topouzian L. Anatomy and physiology of the extensor apparatus of the toes. J Bone Joint Surg 1969;51:669–79.
6. Coughlin M, Mann R. Surgery of the foot and ankle. St. Louis: Mosby; 1999. p. 327.
7. Hagy J, Mann R, Keller C. Gait analysis laboratory, Shriners Hospital, San Francisco: Normal Electromyographic Data; 1973.
8. Kelikian H. Hallux valgus. Allided deformities of the forefoot and metatarsagia. Philadelphia: Saunders; 1965. p. 292.
9. DuVries H. Acquired nontraumatic deformities of the foot. In: Inman VT, editor. DuVries surgery of the foot. 3rd edition. St. Louis: Mosby; 1973. p. 204.
10. Cameron H, Fedorkow D. Revision rates in forefoot surgery. Foot Ankle 1982;3:47–9.
11. Alvine F, Garvin K. Peg and dowel fusion of the proximal interphalangeal joint. Foot Ankle 1980;1:90–4.
12. Coughlin M. Lesser toe deformities. Orthopaedics 1987;10:6–75.
13. Harmonson J, Harkless L. Operative procedures for the correction of hammertoe, claw toe and mallet toe: a literature review. Clin Podiatr Med Surg 1996;13:211–20.

14. Konkel K, Menger A, Retzlaff S. Hammer toe correction using an absorbable intramedullary pin. Foot Ankle Int 2007;28:916–20.
15. Lamm B, Ribeiro C, Valhovic T, et al. Lesser proximal interphalangeal joint arthrodesis: a retrospective analysis of the peg-in-hole and end-to-end procedures. J Am Podiatr Med Assoc 2001;91:331–6.
16. Lehman D, Smith R. Treatment of symptomatic hammertoe with a proximal interphalangeal joint arthrodesis. Foot Ankle Int 1995;16:535–41.
17. Pietrzak W, Lessek T, Perns S. A bioabsorbable fixation implant for use in proximal interphalangeal joint (hammer toe) arthrodesis: biomechanical testing in a synthetic bone substrate. J Foot Ankle Surg 2006;45:288–94.
18. Shaw A, Alvarez G. The use of digital implants for the correction of hammer toe deformity and their potential complications and management. J Foot Surg 1992;31:63–74.
19. Taylor R. The Treatment of claw toes by multiple transfers of flexion into extensor tendons. J Bone Joint Surg 1951;33-B:539–42.
20. Ellington J, Anderson R, Davis W, et al. Radiographic analysis of proximal interphalangeal joint arthrodesis with an intramedullary fusion device for lesser toe deformities. Foot Ankle Int 2010;31:372–6.
21. Kimmel H, Garrow S. A comparison of end-to-end versus "V" arthrodesis procedures for the correction of digital deformities. Clin Podiatr Med Surg 1996;13:239–50.
22. Pichney G, Derner R, Lauf E. Digital "V" arthrodesis. J Foot Ankle Surg 1993;32:473–9.
23. Miller J, Blacklidge D, Ferdowsian V, et al. Chevron arthrodesis of the interphalangeal joint for hammertoe correction. J Foot Ankle Surg 2010;49:194–6.
24. Yu G, Vincer A, Wissam E, et al. Techniques for digital arthrodesis: revisiting the old and discovering the new. Clin Podiatr Med Surg 2004;21:17–50.
25. Edwards W, Beischer A. Interphalangeal joint arthrodesis of the lesser toes. Foot Ankle Clin 2002;7:43–8.
26. Harmonson J, Harkless L. Operative procedures for the correction of hammertoe, claw toe, and mallet toe: a literature review. Clin Podiatr Med Surg 1996;13:211–20.
27. Schelfman B, Fento C, McGlamry E. Peg in hole arthrodesis. J Am Podiatr Assoc 1983;73:187–95.
28. Caterini R, Farsetti P, Tarantino U, et al. Arthrodesis of the toe joints with an intramedullary cannulated screw for correction of hammertoe deformity. Foot Ankle Int 2004;25:256–61.
29. Coughlin M. Lesser toe abnormalities. In: Operative orthopaedics. Philadelphia: Lippincott; 1993. p. 2213–8.
30. McConnell B. Correction of hammer-toe deformity: a 10 year review of subperiosteal waist resection of the proximal phalanx. Orthop Rev 1975;8:65–9.
31. McConnell B. Hammertoe surgery: waist resection of the proximal phalanx, a more simplified procedure. South Med J 1975;68:595–8.
32. Cahill B, Connor D. A long-term follow-up on proximal phalangectomy for hammer toes. Clin Orthop 1972;86:191–2.
33. Conklin M, Smith R. Treatment of the atypical lesser toe deformity with basal hemiphalangectomy. Foot Ankle Int 1994;15:585–94.
34. Daly P, Johnson K. Treatment of painful subluxation or dislocation at the second and third metatarsophalangeal joints by partial proximal phalanx excision and subtotal webbing. Clin Orthop 1992;278:164–70.
35. VanderWilde R, Campbell D. Second toe amputation for chronic painful deformity. Read at the Annual Meeting of the American Orthopaedic Foot and Ankle Society. San Francisco; 1993.
36. Gallentine J, DeOrio J. Removal of the second toe for severe hammertoe deformity in elderly patients. Foot Ankle Int 2005;26:353–8.

Hammertoes/Clawtoes: Metatarsophalangeal Joint Correction

Carolyn Chadwick, MBChB, FRCSEd (Tr&Orth)*,
Terry S. Saxby, MBBS, FRACS (Orth)

KEYWORDS

• Clawtoe • Hammertoe • MTPJ correction

Despite their size and location at the distal extremities, the lesser toes can be a major source of discomfort and pain for patient and surgeon alike, and symptoms may be overlooked or underestimated. Commonly patients present with rather nonspecific symptoms, unable to locate accurately the exact site of pain or disability. Understanding the anatomy and potential pathology is crucial, along with careful history taking and examination, to identify the underlying problem.

Of all foot problems, those involving the lesser toes are most common, with a reported incidence of up to 20%.[1] Lesser toe problems occur more commonly in women,[2] and the incidence rises with advancing age.[3]

There has been some confusion over the years regarding the definition of clawtoes and hammertoes. Various combinations of deformities at the metatarsophalangeal (MTPJ), proximal interphalangeal (PIPJ), and distal interphalangeal (DIPJ) joints have been described, and a recent paper by Schrier and colleagues[1] highlights the confusion in definitions among 101 orthopaedic departments. As defined by Coughlin and Mann and confirmed by others,[1] the distinguishing deformity occurs at the MTPJ, but they are probably manifestations of a spectrum of the same pathologic process. A hammertoe involves flexion of the middle and distal phalanges on the proximal phalanx with no deformity at the MTPJ. A clawtoe has hyperextension at the MTPJ with flexion deformity at the PIPJ. Distinguishing between the two should therefore guide the surgeon to the appropriate treatment; however, in common practice these deformities are frequently grouped together and treated in the same manner.[4,5]

The authors have nothing to disclose.
Brisbane Foot and Ankle Centre, Brisbane Private Hospital, 259 Wickham Terrace, Brisbane, 4000, Australia
* Corresponding author.
E-mail address: chittychadwick@hotmail.com

Foot Ankle Clin N Am 16 (2011) 559–571
doi:10.1016/j.fcl.2011.08.006 **foot.theclinics.com**
1083-7515/11/$ – see front matter

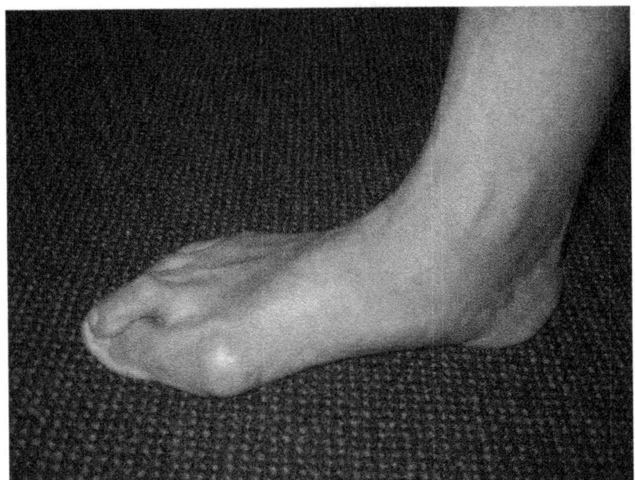

Fig. 1. Clawing of the second toe with associated hallux valgus deformity.

ETIOLOGY AND PATHOPHYSIOLOGY

Several factors contribute to the deformity that is a clawtoe or hammertoe. Constricting footwear causes crowding of the toes and high-heeled footwear leads to forced hyperextension at the MTPJ.[6] It is therefore not surprising that such a number of women encounter problems, as 86% of women wear shoes that are too narrow or too short.[7] An imbalance between the intrinsic flexors and long extensors plays an important role.[8,9] Chronic hyperextension at the MTPJ leads to loss of the tenodesing effect of the long extensor at the PIPJ. The pull of strong extrinsic flexors then creates flexion deformity at the PIPJ.[8] Age-related changes of the soft tissues lead to insufficiency or failure of the plantar plate apparatus, disruption of the plantar capsule, and instability of the MTPJ. The deformity is often associated with hallux valgus (**Fig. 1**). It may be congenital or associated with underlying inflammatory conditions such as rheumatoid or psoriatic arthritis, diabetes, and neuromuscular conditions such as Charcot-Marie-Tooth disease.[3,5] When multiple clawtoes are present, this may indicate an underlying neurologic condition.

CLINICAL EXAMINATION

The foot is examined with the patient standing so that hind foot alignment can be assessed simultaneously. Other findings such as a cavus deformity may indicate an underlying neuromuscular condition. Associated forefoot deformities such as hallux valgus should be identified. The plantar surface is inspected for areas of callosity (**Fig. 2**). With the patient seated, it can be determined whether the lesser toe deformities are fixed or dynamic. As the ankle moves from plantar flexion to dorsiflexion, the toes are seen to claw with a dynamic deformity. Interphalangeal joints are examined for fixed or flexible deformity.

NONOPERATIVE TREATMENT

Treatment can be nonoperative, with footwear advice regarding shoes with a wide toe box and flat heel and shoes made of material with a soft upper and padding beneath.

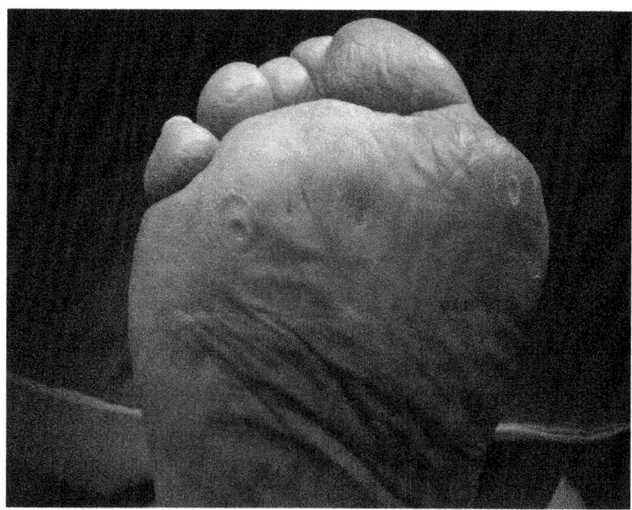

Fig. 2. Multiple painful plantar callosities in a patient with hallux valgus and clawing of the lesser toes.

Taping and the use of nonsteroidal anti-inflammatory drugs (NSAIDs) are also advocated.[3] A cortisone injection may improve associated swelling and synovitis at the MTPJ. A padded insert or metatarsal dome may help symptoms of metatarsalgia. Once the MTPJ becomes subluxed or dislocated, surgery should be considered to prevent further deterioration and development of fixed deformity. Commonly, a hallux valgus deformity may also be present. This may be the cause of, or developed secondarily to, lesser toe deformity. The hallux deformity should ideally be addressed at the time of lesser toe correction to provide space for the corrected second toe.[3] If procedures are to be performed at both the MTPJ and PIPJ, then careful attention must be paid to the neurovascular status as these may well be impaired by stretching or repeated procedures.

OPERATIVE TREATMENT

Multiple procedures for the correction of such deformities are described. This article discusses options of correction at the MTPJ, which can be divided into soft-tissue, bony, and joint ablation procedures.

Soft-Tissue Procedures

Following a cadaveric model investigating the anatomy of clawtoes and hammertoes by Myerson and Sherreff in 1989,[10] Dhukaram and coworkers retrospectively reviewed 179 hammertoes treated with an extended release of the MTPJ and PIPJ arthrodesis.[5] With regard to the MTPJ, the position of the toe was assessed with the ankle in neutral dorsiflexion at each step of the release. When satisfactory toe alignment was achieved, and the plantar fat pad was reduced, no further release was required. The sequence of release was as follows: Z-lengthening or release of the extensor digitorum longus, division of the extensor digitorum brevis, dorsal capsule release, collateral ligament release, mobilization, and reduction of the plantar plate (**Fig. 3**). If extension remained at the MTPJ, a Weil metatarsal osteotomy was

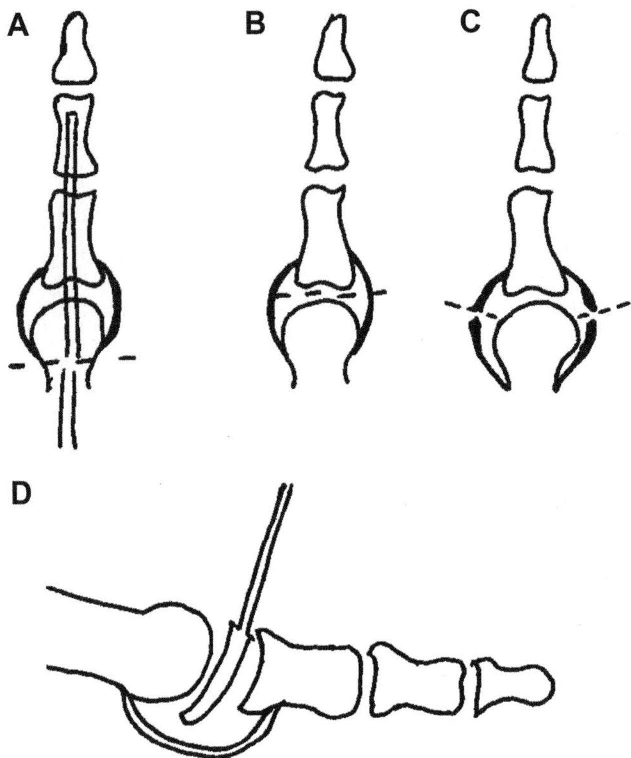

Fig. 3. AP view showing stepwise soft tissue release of (*A*) extensor digitorum brevis, (*B*) MTPJ capsule, (*C*) collateral ligaments, and (*D*) lateral view showing a blunt curved instrument to reduce the plantar plate under the metatarsal head.

performed, followed by flexor-to-extensor transfer for further stabilization of the MTPJ.[5] Dhukaram and coworkers showed good results, with an average American Orthopaedic Foot and Ankle Society (AOFAS) score of 83. The main reason for poor outcome was the incidence of pain at the MTPJ joint, and to a lesser degree, excessive release leading to floppiness and pain under the tip of the toe.

With flexible hammertoes or clawtoes, the foot may appear normal with the patient sitting and the ankle in equinus, thus relaxing the extrinsic flexor tendons. On weight bearing, as the ankle is brought into a neutral or dorsiflexed position, the toes appear to claw, due to contraction of the flexor tendons. Although a tenotomy will correct deformity at the PIPJ, this alone will not address the MTPJ hyperextension and therefore a flexor-to-extensor transfer may be necessary to hold the proximal phalanx in a neutral position, substituting the loss of intrinsic function.[11]

The flexor-to-extensor transfer has been described by many authors.[3,9,12] There have been minor modifications described by others more recently.[11,13] The procedure involves a plantar transverse incision at the MTPJ and identification of the flexor digitorum longus (FDL) tendon by its median raphe. The tendon is released distally through a separate stab incision at the DIPJ and delivered into the proximal wound and split longitudinally. Each limb is then routed subcutaneously to the dorsum of the proximal phalanx into the extensor hood and the toe further stabilized with a temporary 1.1 mm k-wire with the toe in 20° to 30° flexion and the ankle in neutral.[4]

Postoperatively a soft dressing is applied and the patient can mobilize in a stiff-soled postoperative shoe. The wire is removed at 4 weeks and the toe is taped in a few degrees plantar flexion for a further 4 weeks.

Many authors have published results of flexor-to-extensor tendon transfer results with good results, high patient satisfaction, and few complications.[11,13–15] Boyer and colleagues reviewed 38 patients with 79 affected toes with a mean follow-up of 33 months.[11] Patients with both flexible and fixed PIPJ deformity were treated, most of whom underwent concurrent procedures on the same foot. Patients with a fixed deformity who also had a PIPJ fusion had a better outcome than those with a flexible deformity who did not, although the overall subjective satisfaction rate was high, with 89% of patients willing to have the same procedure again. Of those unsatisfied with their outcome, a common complaint was inability to fit into shoes. There was a higher level of dissatisfaction in patients who underwent concurrent foot procedures at the time of lesser toe correction, and this outcome has also been noted by others.[9,16]

With a fixed flexion deformity of the PIPJ and coexisting deformity at the MTPJ, this must be addressed as well to ensure adequate correction. For mild MTPJ subluxation, a sequential soft-tissue release can be performed, checking for reduction and stability at each stage. Using a dorsal approach the extensor tendons are either Z-lengthened or released completely. A dorsal capsulotomy is performed followed by medial and lateral collateral release. The medial lumbrical is sometimes a significant deforming force on the second MTPJ and therefore requires release if medial deviation as well as dorsal subluxation is observed. With chronic cases where plantar plate adhesions are present, release from the plantar metatarsal head allows adequate reduction of the MTPJ joint. The surgeon should ensure that the toe sits in a reduced position after the soft-tissue release. Some authors advocate the use of a 1.1 mm k-wire across the joint to hold the position for 3 to 4 weeks[11] but should not rely on the k-wire to correct any residual deformity, as removing the wire will lead to recurrent deformity. Results of surgery are generally good, although there are no randomized controlled trials comparing one form of treatment with another.

Vaseenon and colleagues reported on a soft tissue technique in a subgroup of patients with clawtoes secondary to extrinsic pull from a tendinous interconnection to flexor hallucis longus.[17] This is apparent clinically by active flexion against resistance of the hallux, which in turn causes clawing of the lesser toes. By dividing the tendinous interconnection and thus preserving the tendon of FDL, clawing is improved without loss of the grasping function noted with flexor tenotomy.

Bony Procedures

When deformity at the MTPJ is severe with subluxation or dislocation of the proximal phalanx, soft-tissue release alone may not be enough to achieve satisfactory correction and osseous decompression is required. This can be in the form of a shortening osteotomy of the metatarsal head, partial proximal phalangectomy, or arthroplasty of the metatarsal head.

Metatarsal Shortening Osteotomy

Clawtoes and hammertoes are a common cause of metatarsalgia, characterized by severe pain in the region of the metatarsal heads and intractable plantar keratosis. Symptoms occur due to increased downward force of the metatarsal head, a reduction in plantar soft tissue padding, or a combination of both. Distal metatarsal shortening osteotomies aim to relieve plantar pressure and reduce the hyperextended or dislocated MTPJ seen with clawtoes. The following brief overview explains their role in the approach to MTPJ deformity.

An oblique distal metatarsal osteotomy was described by Helal in 1975[18] that allows dorsal and proximal migration of the head, thus shortening the metatarsal, but does not address the contracted soft tissues around the MTPJ. No fixation is used; therefore the distal metatarsal may rest in an unpredictable position. Helal reported 88% good or excellent results using this technique, but less favorable results are reported by others, who in particular note the problem of transfer metatarsalgia.[19,20]

Weil described a distal metatarsal osteotomy through the head and neck, cut parallel to the weight-bearing surface of the foot.[21] This shortening osteotomy axially decompresses the MTPJ as the head slides proximally. The large surface area created by the oblique osteotomy minimizes the risk of non-union, and along with rigid screw fixation, allows for early weight bearing.

Good results using the Weil osteotomy for relieving metatarsalgia caused by deformity at the MTPJ are reported.[22–25] Although the joint is preserved, there are recognized problems with joint stiffness, dorsiflexion contracture at the MTPJ, transfer metatarsalgia, toe weakness, and floating toes.[22–24,26–29]

Modifications of this procedure are described on sawbone models to try and eliminate the problem of plantar displacement of the metatarsal head. Such plantar displacement can lead to a change in the center of rotation of the metatarsal head and subsequent dorsiflexion contracture at the MTPJ along with recurrent metatarsalgia.[30] By altering the angle of the osteotomy which begins proximal to the metatarsal head and resecting a slice or wedge of bone, it is theorized that proximal shift of the metatarsal head is still achieved but plantar displacement is avoided. A retrospective case study of 48 patients (71 feet) treated with segmental osteotomy showed overall outcomes similar to those of other published reports of treatment using the Weil osteotomy.[28] Although there was no difference in complications either, they conclude that the procedure is technically easier to perform. There are, however, no randomized controlled trials to confirm this.

The Weil osteotomy is an effective and reliable surgical option for the treatment of metatarsalgia secondary to clawtoes and hammertoes when nonoperative management has failed, and in the absence of significant inflammatory or erosive arthropathy.

Partial Proximal Hemiphalangectomy

With severe deformity in the presence of joint destruction, salvage options include partial proximal hemiphalangectomy or excision of the metatarsal heads. Partial proximal hemiphalangectomy involves excising the base of the proximal phalanx. If adjacent toes are involved, through a web-based incision hemiphalangectomies may be performed, along with syndactilization.

Daly and Johnson reported 75% of patients (60 feet) were satisfied or satisfied with minor reservations, with the most improvement noted for pain.[31] Conklin reported less favorable results in 86 feet, with 29% of patients dissatisfied, mostly due to persistent flexion deformity at the PIPJ.[32] They also noted that preoperative diagnosis significantly affected outcome. Patients with rheumatoid deformities were more satisfied than those treated for hammertoes or MTPJ subluxation or dislocation from other causes. This may just be reflective of patients with lower functional demand. Cahill reported good relief of symptoms but poor objective outcome and poor cosmetic results.[33] The main complications reported are cock-up deformity, excessive shortening of the toe, and residual pain.[31]

Forefoot Arthroplasty

Severe clawing involving all of the lesser toes is most commonly seen in patients with rheumatoid arthritis, as well as neuromuscular disorders and after trauma. There is often coexisting pathology affecting the first MTPJ as well that must be addressed.

In 1912 Hoffman described a surgical method for treating severe rigid claw deformity with associated plantar pain and callosity under the lesser metatarsal heads.[34] This involved a curved plantar incision and resection of the lesser metatarsal heads. Clayton[35] excised both bases of proximal phalanges and metatarsal heads through a dorsal transverse incision. In 1959 Fowler used a dorsal transverse incision with perpendicular extensions over the first and fifth metatarsals to resect the base of the proximal phalanges as well as trimming the metatarsal heads.[36] An ellipse of plantar skin was also excised to plantar flex the toes and aid relocation of the fat pad more proximally. In 1967, Kates, Kessel, and Kay modified the procedure.[37] Utilizing only a plantar incision, along with excision of an ellipse of skin, all the metatarsal heads are resected, with the remaining metatarsals forming a shallow, smooth arc to prevent further painful pressure areas. Lipscomb in 1968 excised the proximal phalanges and plantar metatarsal condyles through two separate dorsal longitudinal incisions, in combination with extensor tenotomies to the lesser toes, and a Keller procedure for the hallux.[38]

Many authors have published the results of forefoot arthroplasty with generally good subjective results[37–40] (**Fig. 4**). Barton reviewed 65 feet treated with a variety of forefoot arthroplasty techniques as mentioned above.[39] Fifty-two feet (80%) had mild or no pain postoperatively, although a third of those examined still had plantar prominence of the metatarsal heads. Stockley and colleagues reported 70% of patients were pain free 3 years after a Kates, Kessel, Kay procedure[41]; however, others showed less pain relief, in particular one long-term study reporting more than 50% of patients were dissatisfied due to pain.[42] Recurrent plantar callosity is commonly recognized by others too.[40] Van der Heijden reported a 25% reoperation rate for this problem in 16 feet of 10 patients.[43] In Barton's paper,[39] 63 of 65 feet were reported subjectively as a successful outcome, with minor reservations including some pain, poor balance, and unequal foot size. Objective outcomes were less favorable. There were a significant number of problems with wound healing, occurring in more than one third of operated feet, irrespective of which approach was used. Other rates of wound healing problems with the plantar approach have been reported as 8%[43] and 13%.[44] Objective function was also poor with regard to useful toe function and gait.

The treatment of multiple clawed toes in the rheumatoid forefoot is a far more complex problem than that of an isolated clawtoe, due to the coexisting abnormality at the first MTPJ. Coughlin and coworkers, in their long-term follow-up study, highlighted the importance of achieving a stable realigned first ray to prevent stressing the lateral MTPJs and recurrence of plantar callosity and pain.[40] Other studies, however, showed no significant difference in clinical outcome, comparing arthrodesis with excision arthroplasty of the hallux MTPJ.[45,46] Thordarson found an 85% failure rate with surgery for the rheumatoid forefoot that preserved the hallux MTPJ.[47] Other studies have shown a higher reoperation rate in patients undergoing excision arthroplasty of the first MTPJ.[40,48]

There is difficulty comparing the outcomes of forefoot arthroplasty, as many studies predate the introduction of the AOFAS standardized scoring system in 1994.[49] In one recent long-term follow-up of the modified Hoffman procedure, all 20 patients (37 feet) were satisfied with the results of surgery, with 4 wound problems but no reoperations.[50] They compared their results with those of Mann and Thompson in

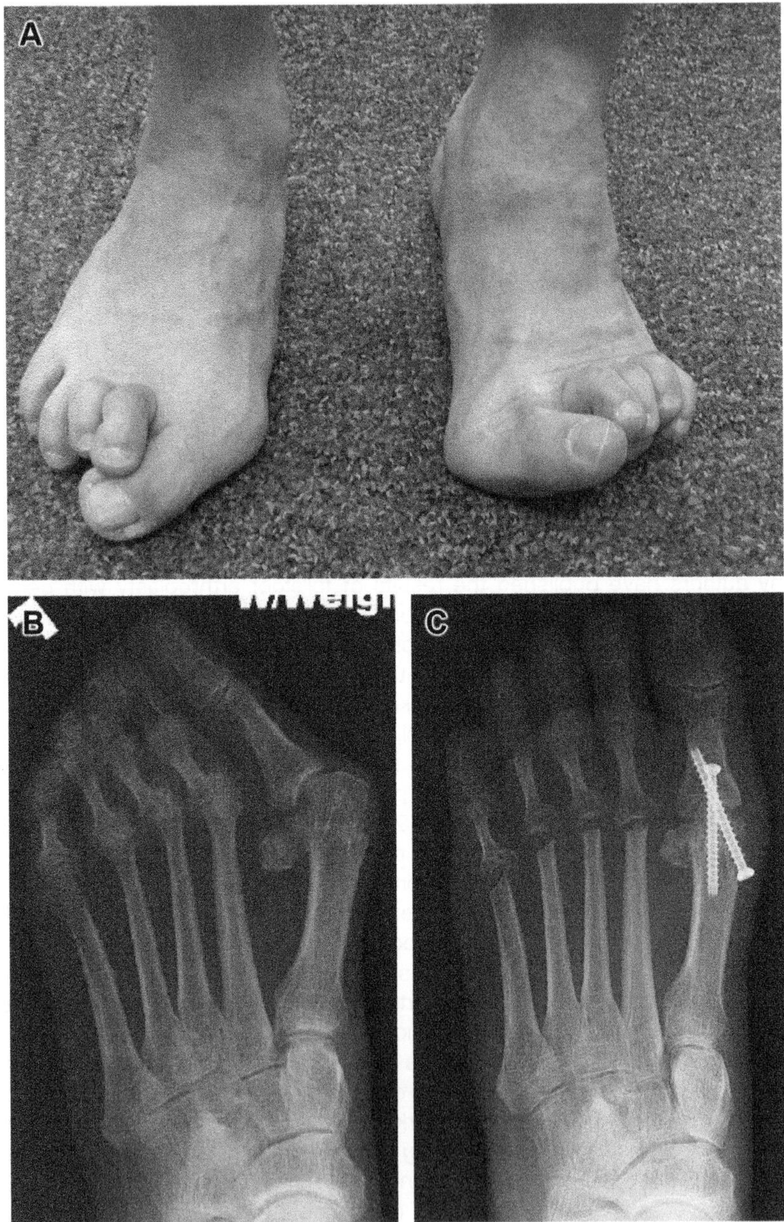

Fig. 4. (*A*) Severe hallux valgus and multiple clawed toes. (*B, C*) Preoperative and postoperative radiographs after excision arthroplasty of the lesser metatarsal heads and arthrodesis of the first MTPJ.

1984[51] and Coughlin in 2000.[40] Comparison with Thompson's paper was made using strict criteria, as defined by Thompson, based on the visual analogue score and pain when walking. Thompson's 89% good or excellent results were far superior to the 30% noted in the more recent study, most likely due to the criterion that any pain at all was deemed a fair or poor result. Subjective results, however, were much the same. Comparison with Coughlin's paper revealed the AOFAS score was similar (64.5 compared with 69), but in that study, the first MTPJ was fused rather than excised, and given the polyarticular nature of rheumatoid arthritis it is difficult to attribute pain or poor function to one joint or another.

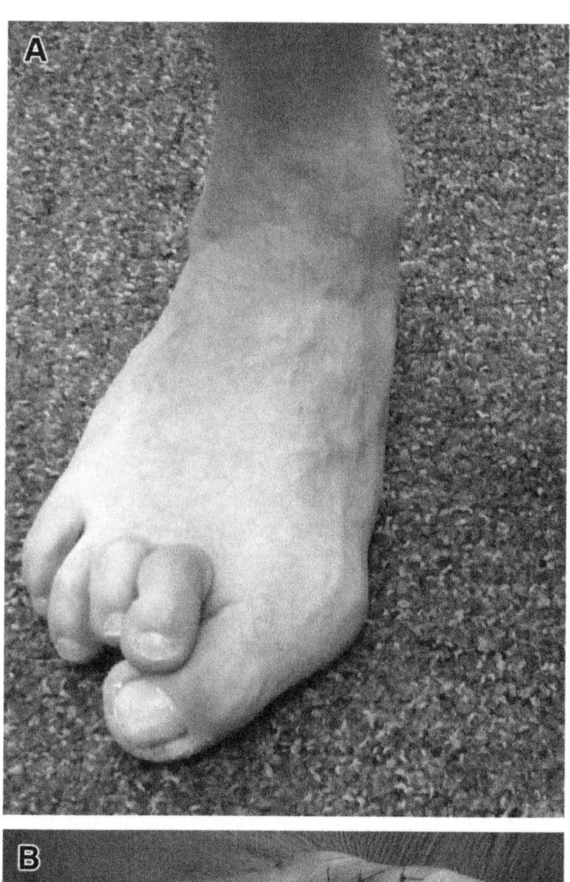

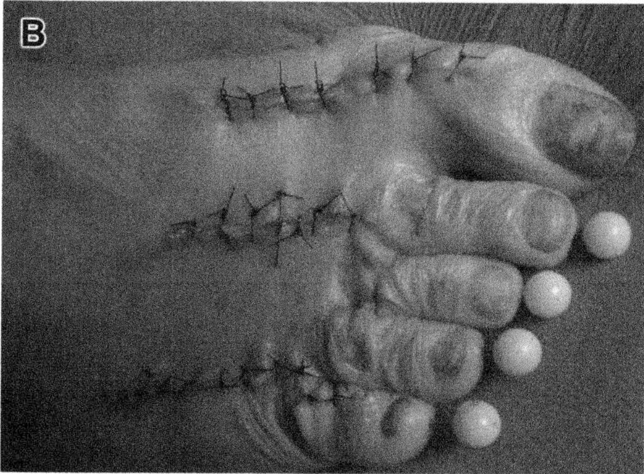

Fig. 5. (*A*) Patient with rheumatoid arthritis with hallux valgus and clawtoes. (*B*) After first MTPJ fusion, forefoot arthroplasty, and PIPJ fusions.

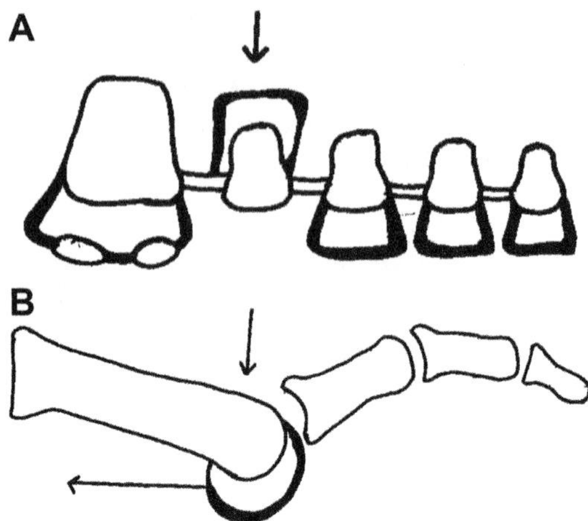

Fig. 6. The plunger effect. (*A*) Coronal view showing the displaced plantar plate in a dorsal position as the toe claws. By its attachment to the transverse metatarsal ligament, the plantar plate creates a dorsoplantar force, depressing the metatarsal (MT) head. (*B*) Sagittal view. The plantar fascia is displaced along with the stretched plantar plate. On weight bearing, the fascia tightens and the MT head is depressed further.

Regarding the associated flexion deformity at the PIPJ, treatment depends on the degree of severity. Treatments include simple manipulation, proximal phalanx condylectomy, and interphalangeal fusion.[40] Without adequate realignment of the PIPJ, the proximal phalanx remains in a hyperextended position, increasing the possibility of recurrent callosity and deformity.[40]

Despite the less favorable functional results reported, the subjective results justify surgery in a group of patients with low functional demand, disabled by severe pain (**Fig. 5**).

Another method of forefoot arthroplasty, preserving the metatarsal heads, has been described Briggs and Stainsby.[52] They initially recognized the importance of the plantar plate and its attachment to the deep transverse metatarsal ligament and plantar aponeurosis, which when displaced dorsally as the proximal phalanx subluxes or dislocates, causes metatarsal head depression due to the so-called "plunger" effect[53] (**Fig. 6**). The approach in treating both isolated and multiple clawtoe deformities, as in the rheumatoid foot, emphasizes the importance of relocation of the plantar plate underneath the metatarsal head and thus the function of the plantar fat pad. Through a dorsal angled incision, the extensor tendon is divided, the base of the proximal phalanx is excised, the plantar plate is freed and repositioned under the metatarsal head. The toe is stabilized with a wire across the MTPJ and the distal stump of the extensor tendon is sutured to the flexor tendon. This latter step of extensor-to-flexor tenodesis is not performed by all.

Results at an average 40-month follow-up showed 83% of single toes operated on (69 feet) had a good or excellent subjective outcome, and 74% had satisfactory objective outcome with reason for poor satisfaction being metatarsalgia, recurrent callosity, and recurrent MTPJ dislocation. Those who had multiple lesser toes treated as part of rheumatoid forefoot correction showed a 93% good or excellent subjective outcome. Complications were minimal, with minor wound problems being the most common. Subsequent studies have shown equally good functional results, although cosmetic outcome is not so favorable.[54–56]

Amputation

In cases of isolated symptomatic hammertoes associated with other asymptomatic forefoot abnormalities, amputation through the MTPJ is a reasonable option to reduce the morbidity associated with complex forefoot reconstruction. Gallentine[57] retrospectively reviewed 12 elderly patients with painful second hammertoes, of whom 10 were satisfied and 2 satisfied with reservations. This is a simple and valid method of treating focal pain from a severe hammertoe deformity that avoids extensive surgery elsewhere in the foot.

SUMMARY

Clawing of the lesser toes is not uncommon, can arise from a number of causes, and is often associated with other forefoot abnormalities. There is still some confusion in the nomenclature of lesser toe deformities affecting the MTPJ and PIPJ although the resulting deformities are probably part of the same pathologic process and thus treated in a similar manner. Many will be successfully treated with nonoperative methods, but if they fail a number of surgical options are available depending on the severity of the deformity and whether the deformity is fixed or flexible. Correction at the MTPJ can be achieved using a stepwise progression of soft-tissue procedures alone, bony procedures, or a combination of both.

REFERENCES

1. Schrier JC, Louwerens JW, Verheyen CC. Opinions on lesser toe deformities among Dutch orthopaedic departments. Foot Ankle Int 2007;28(12):1265–70.
2. Femino JE, Mueller K. Complications of lesser toe surgery. Clin Orthop Relat Res 2001;391:72–88.
3. Coughlin MJ. Lesser toe abnormalities. An Instructional course lecture. American Academy of Orthopaedic Surgeons. J Bone Joint Surg Am 2002;84A(8):1446–69.
4. Coughlin MJ. Subluxation and dislocation of the second metatarsophalangeal joint. Orthop Clin North Am 1989;20(4):535–51.
5. Dhukaram V, Hossain S, Sampath J, Barrie JL. Correction of hammer-toe with an extended release of the metatarsophalangeal joint. J Bone Joint Surg Br 2002;84(7): 986–90.
6. Coughlin MJ. Mallet toes, hammer toes, claw toes, and corns. Causes and treatment of lesser-toe deformities. Postgrad Med 1984;75(5):191–8.
7. Frey C, Thompson F, Smith J. Update on women's footwear. Foot Ankle Int 1995; 16(6):328–31.
8. Scheck M. Etiology of acquired hammer-toe deformity. Clin Orthop Relat Res 1977; 123:63–9.
9. Pyper JB. The flexor-extensor transplant operation for claw toes. J Bone Joint Surge Br 1958;40-B(3):528–33.
10. Myerson MS, Sherreff MJ. The pathological anatomy of claw and hammer-toes. J Bone Joint Surg Am 1989;71-A:45–9.
11. Boyer ML, DeOrio JK. Transfer of the flexor digitorum longus for the correction of lesser toe deformities. Foot Ankle Int 2007;28(4):422–30.
12. Taylor RG. The treatment of claw toes by multiple transfers of flexor into extensor tendons. J Bone Joint Surg Br 1951;33-B(4):539–42.
13. Kuwada GT. A retrospective analysis of modification of the flexor tendon transfer for correction of hammertoes. J Foot Surg 1988;5:57–9.
14. Barbari SG, Brevig K. Correction of claw toes by the Girdlestone-Taylor flexor-extensor transfer procedure. Foot Ankle 1984;5:67–73.

15. Parrish TF. Dynamic correction of clawtoes. Orthop Clin North Am 1973;4(1):97–102.
16. Coughlin MJ, Dorris J, Polk E. Operative repair of the fixed hammertoe deformity. Foot Ankle Int 2000;21(2):94–104.
17. Vaseenon T, Phisitkul P. A novel tendinous interconnection release technique for claw toe deformity. Iowa Orthop J 2010;30:157–60.
18. Helal B. Metatarsal osteotomy for metatarsalgia. J Bone Joint Surg 1975;57(2): 187–92.
19. Trnka HJ, Muhlbauer M, Zettl R. Comparison of the results of the Weil and the Helal osteotomies for the treatment of metatarsalgia secondary to dislocation of the lesser MTPJs. Foot Ankle Int 1999;20:72–9.
20. Trnka HJ, Kabon B, Zettl R, et al. Helal metatarsal osteotomy for the treatment a critical analysis of results. Orthopedics 1996;19(5):457–61.
21. Barouk LS. Weil's metatarsal osteotomy in the treatment of metatarsalgia. Orthopade 1996;25(4):338–44.
22. Trnka HJ, Gebhard C, Muhlbauer M. The Weil osteotomy for the treatment of dislocated lesser MTPJs. Acta Orthop Scand 2002;73:190–4.
23. Hofstaetter SG, Hoffstaetter JG. The Weil osteotomy. A 7 year follow up. J Bone Joint Surg Br 2005;87(7):1507–11.
24. Vandeputte G, Deremarker G, Steenwercks A, et al. The Weil osteotomy of the lesser metatarsals: a clinical and pedobarographic follow-up study. Foot Ankle Int 2000;21: 370–4.
25. Davies MS, Saxby TS. Metatarsal neck osteotomy with rigid internal fixation for the treatment of lesser toe metatarsophalangeal joint pathology. Foot Ankle Int 1999; 20(10):630–5.
26. Trnka HJ, Nyska M, Parks BG, et al. Dorsiflexion contracture after the Weil osteotomy: results of a cadaver study and three dimensional analysis. Foot Ankle Int 2001;22: 47–50.
27. Migues A, Slullitel G, Bilbao F, et al. Floating toe deformity as a complication of the Weil osteotomy. Foot Ankle Int 2004;25(9):609–13.
28. Garg R, Thordarson DB, Schrumpf M, et al. Sliding oblique versus segmental resection osteotomies for lesser metatarsophalangeal joint pathology. Foot Ankle Int 2008;29(10):1009–14.
29. Beech I, Rees S, Tagoe MJ. A retrospective review of the Weil osteotomy for lesser metatarsal deformities: an intermediate follow-up analysis. Foot Ankle Surg 2005; 44(5):358–64.
30. Melamed EA, Schon LC, Myerson MS. 2 modifications of the Weil osteotomy: analysis on sawbone models. Foot Ankle Int 2002;23(5):400–5.
31. Daly PJ, Johnson KA. Treatment of painful subluxation or dislocation at the second and third metatarsophalangeal joints by partial proximal phalanx excision and subtotal webbing. Clin Orthop Relat Res 1992;(278):164–70.
32. Conklin MJ, Smith RW. Treatment of the atypical lesser toe deformity with basal hemiphalangectomy. Foot Ankle Int 1994;15(11):585–94.
33. Cahill BR, Connor DE. A long-term follow-up on proximal phalangectomy for hammer toes. Clin Orthop 1972;86:191–2.
34. Hoffman P. An operation for severe grades of contracted or claw toes. Am J Orthop Surg 1912;9;441–9.
35. Clayton ML. Surgery of the forefoot in rheumatoid arthritis. Clin Orthop Relat Res 1960;16:136–40.
36. Fowler AW. A method of forefoot reconstruction. J Bone Joint Surg Br 1959;41-B: 507–13.

37. Kates A, Kessel L, Kay A. Arthroplasty of the forefoot. J Bone Joint Surg Br 1967;49:552–7.
38. Lipscomb PR. Surgery for rheumatoid arthritis-timing and techniques: summary. J Bone Joint Surg Am 1968;50(3):614–7.
39. Barton NJ. Arthroplasty of the forefoot in rheumatoid arthritis. J Bone Joint Surg Br 1973;55(1):126–33.
40. Coughlin MJ. Rheumatoid forefoot reconstruction. A long-term follow-up study. J Bone Joint Surg Am 2000;82(3):322–41.
41. Stockley I, Betts RP, Getty CJ, et al. A prospective study of forefoot arthroplasty. Clin Orthop Relat Res 1989;248:213–8.
42. Patsalis T, Georgousis H, Göpfert S. Long-term results of forefoot arthroplasty in patients with rheumatoid arthritis. Orthopedics 1996;19(5):439–47.
43. van der Heijden KW, Rasker JJ, Jacobs JW, et al. Kates forefoot arthroplasty in rheumatoid arthritis. A 5-year followup study. Rheumatology 1992;19(10):1545–50.
44. Faithful DK, Savill DL. Review of the results of excision of the metatarsal heads in patients with rheumatoid arthritis. Ann Rheum Dis 1971;30(2):201–2.
45. Beauchamp CG, Kirby T, Rudge SR, et al. Fusion of the first metatarsophalangeal joint in forefoot arthroplasty. Clin Orthop Relat Res 1984;190:249–53.
46. Hughes J, Grace D, Clark P, et al. Metatarsal head excision for rheumatoid arthritis. 4-year follow-up of 68 feet with and without hallux fusion. Acta Orthop Scand 199;62(1):63–6.
47. Thordarson DB, Aval S, Krieger L. Failure of hallux MP preservation surgery for rheumatoid arthritis. Foot Ankle Int 2002;23(6):486–90.
48. Hulse N, Thomas AM. Metatarsal head resection in the rheumatoid foot: 5–year follow-up with and without resection of the first metatarsal head. J Foot Ankle Surg 2006;45(2):107–12.
49. Kitaoka HB, Alexander IJ, Adelaar RS, et al. Clinical rating systems for the ankle-hindfoot, midfoot, hallux and lesser-toes. Foot Ankle Int 1994;15(7):349–53.
50. Thomas S, Kinninmonth AW, Kumar CS. Long-term results of the modified Hoffman procedure in the rheumatoid foot. J Bone Joint Surg Am 2005;87(4):748–52.
51. Mann RA, Thompson FM. Arthrodesis of the first metatarsophalangeal joint for hallux valgus in rheumatoid arthritis. J Bone Joint Surg Am 1984;66(5):687–92.
52. Briggs PJ, Stainsby GD. Metatarsal head preservation in forefoot arthroplasty and the correction of severe claw toe deformity. Foot Ankle 2001;7:93–101.
53. Stainsby GD. Pathological anatomy and dynamic effect of the displaced plantar plate and the importance of the plantar plate-deep transverse metatarsal ligament tie–bar. Ann R Coll Surg Eng 1997;79:58–68.
54. Hossain S. Stainsby procedure for non-rheumatoid claw toes. Foot Ankle Surg 2003;9:113–8.
55. Queally JM, Zgraj OS, Walsh JC, et al. Use of the modified Stainsby procedure in correcting severe claw toe deformity in the rheumatoid foot: a retrospective review. The Foot 2009;19(2):110–3.
56. Hassana K, Rashida MA, Panikkara V. Forefoot reconstruction: effectiveness of Stainsby operation in treating disclocated lesser toes. The Foot 2007;17(3):136–42.
57. Gallentine JW, DeOrio JK. Removal of the second toe for severe hammer-toe deformity in elderly patients. Foot Ankle Int 2005;26:353–8.

The Use of Flexor to Extensor Transfers for the Correction of the Flexible Hammer Toe Deformity

John Y. Kwon, MD[a,b,*], Richard J. De Asla, MD[a,b]

KEYWORDS

• Hammer toe • Clawtoe • Flexion deformity • Foot

Hammer toes are flexion deformities of the proximal interphalangeal (PIP) joint and are often associated with ill-fitting shoe wear. Less commonly they can be attributed to congenital and neuromuscular conditions.[1–4] Multiple factors contribute to the development of this deformity, but prevalence is higher in women and with advanced age.[5–9] The dorsal aspect of the PIP joint is most commonly painful because of pressure or shearing within the toe box of the shoe (**Fig. 1**). Pain at the distal-most aspect of the toe may also occur from rubbing against the insole. More severe deformities may hinder the plantar flexion power of the toe, resulting in metatarsalgia. Patients with peripheral neuropathy are at increased risk for ulcer formation over the dorsal PIP joint and distal toe.

A hammer toe is characterized by a PIP flexion deformity without significant abnormality at the distal interphalangeal (DIP) joint. There is typically no to mild extension deformity of the metatarsophalangeal (MTP) joint. A clawtoe is characterized by hyperextension at the MTP joint, flexion at the PIP joint, and often a flexion deformity at the DIP joint. However, the terms *hammer toe* and *clawtoe* have often been interchangeable in the literature.

PATHOPHYSIOLOGY

The underlying pathophysiology that results in hammer toe deformity involves a disruption of the complex balance between toe extensors and flexors, as well as weakening of the static restraints of the toe including the plantar plate and collateral ligaments. The extensor digitorum longus (EDL) is the extrinsic extensor to the toe and possesses several attachments. A middle slip attaches onto the base of the middle

[a] Foot & Ankle Division, Department of Orthopaedic Surgery, Massachusetts General Hospital, 55 Fruit Street, Boston, MA 02114, USA
[b] Harvard Medical School, 25 Shattuck Street, Boston, MA 02115, USA
* Corresponding author.
E-mail address: johnkwonmd@gmail.com

Foot Ankle Clin N Am 16 (2011) 573–582
doi:10.1016/j.fcl.2011.08.005
foot.theclinics.com
1083-7515/11/$ – see front matter

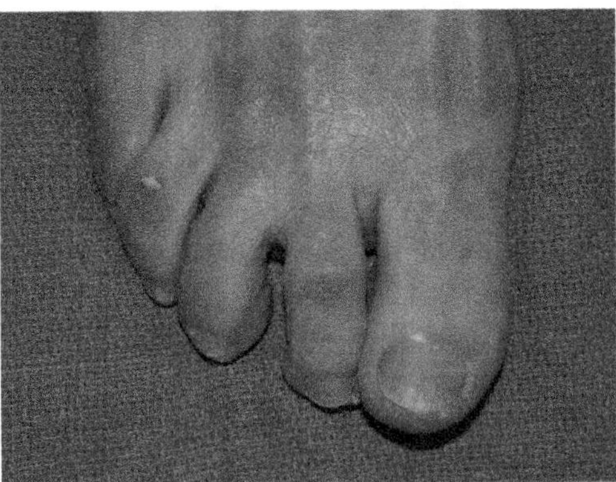

Fig. 1. Multiple hammer toes with dorsal PIP irritation of the second and fourth toes.

phalanx, whereas two lateral slips extend distally and converge to attach to the base of the distal phalanx. Although there is no insertion on the proximal phalanx per se, the EDL functions to dorsiflex the proximal phalanx via attachments to the extensor hood and distal phalanges. The flexor digitorum longus (FDL) attaches to the plantar aspect of the distal phalanx, whereas the flexor digitorum brevis (FDB) attaches to the plantar aspect of the middle phalanx. The former causes flexion at both the DIP and PIP joints whereas the later causes flexion at the PIP joint. As with the extensors, there is no direct flexor attachment to the proximal phalanx. However, unlike the dorsal structures, there is no aponeurotic sling to provide significant isolated flexion at the MTP joint.

The lumbricals and interossei are the intrinsic muscles to the foot and function in a similar way to those found in the hand. The lumbricals are situated plantar to the transverse metatarsal ligament, and the interossei are dorsal. Both pass plantar to the MTP joint center of rotation and dorsal to the PIP and DIP centers of rotation. The result is flexion at the MTP joint and simultaneous extension of both interphalangeal (IP) joints. As dorsiflexion at the MTP joint increases, the ability of the intrinsics to counter the resultant toe deformity lessens secondary to an alteration in their line of pull.

The plantar plate, joint capsules, and collateral ligaments are the static toe stabilizers. The plantar plate inserts from the plantar neck of the metatarsal to the plantar base of the proximal phalanx and is a major contributor to MTP joint stability. Furthermore, the plantar plate functions as a central stabilizer to the FDL, which courses directly plantar to it. Whether attenuated by repetitive strain or injured acutely, the plantar plate's ability to limit hyperdorsiflexion at the MTP joint can become compromised. Fortin and Myerson[10] demonstrated in a cadaver study that sectioning the plantar plate resulted in 29% less force required to dislocate this joint. Haddad and colleagues[11] demonstrated that the weakest portion of the joint capsule was the synovial attachment of the plantar plate to the metatarsal neck.

The MTP joint collateral ligaments are made up of two components: the phalangeal collateral ligaments that insert on the proximal phalanx and the accessory collateral ligaments that insert on the plantar plate. These ligaments are the primary stabilizers of the lesser MTP joint, with cadaver studies showing 48% less force required to dislocate these joints when sectioned.[10]

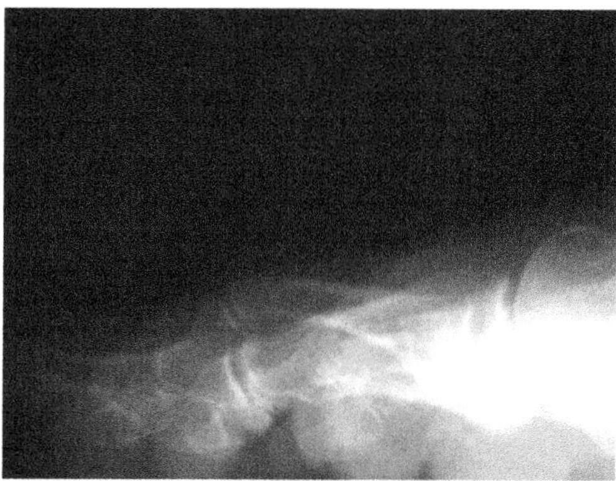

Fig. 2. Lateral view of hammer toe deformity.

Repetitive external deforming forces can potentiate both attenuation of static structures and alter dynamic stabilizer balance. Chronic unbalanced dynamic forces may also attenuate static stabilizers and ultimately result in toe deformity. A common example of such a scenario is found in narrow high-heeled shoes. A cramped toe box limits toe motion, and in time intrinsic weakness follows. The constant dorsiflexed posture that the MTP joint assumes attenuates the plantar plate. With reduced ability to limit proximal phalangeal translation, dorsal subluxation of the proximal phalanx on the metatarsal head occurs. Compensatory shortening and contracture of the EDL follows, which diminishes its ability to extend the IP joints. In addition, dorsiflexion at the MTP joint similarly reduces the ability of the lumbricals and interossei to maintain adequate MTP flexion and IP extension moments as relationships between the various force vectors to their respective joint axes change. The dorsiflexed proximal phalanx effectively tensions the FDL and FDB that in turn overpower the already weakened intrinsics. The attenuated plantar plate may also allow the FDL tendon to subluxate, altering its force vector and exacerbating deformity.

EVALUATION

Physical examination is critical to guide treatment, especially if surgery is to be considered. Careful examination of the foot and ankle should be performed not only to assess the toes, but also to identify other possible causes for the hammer toe deformity. Inspection is performed to assess overall foot posture and identify callosities or corns indicating areas of pressure. Passive and active range of motion at all joints (including the ankle to look for Achilles contractures), strength, and neurovascular status are evaluated. Assessing toe perfusion and overall vascular status of the foot is of particular importance prior to considering any surgical intervention. Alignment should be assessed in the sagittal plane as well as for medial or lateral deviation. Noting the degree of flexibility at the MTP, PIP, and DIP joints is critical because surgical treatment for rigid deformity is different than for flexible deformity. In addition to clinical examination, radiographic examination is important to further assess deformity and the presence of arthritis or other osseous conditions. Weight bearing may accentuate certain deformities, and therefore weight bearing radiographs are preferred (**Fig. 2**).

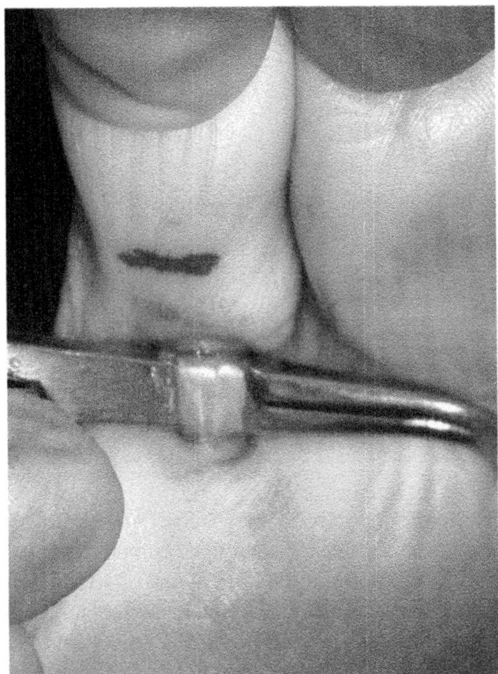

Fig. 3. Hemostat placed underneath both flexor tendons.

NONOPERATIVE TREATMENT AND SURGICAL INDICATIONS

Initial nonsurgical treatment is recommended for symptomatic hammer toes in most cases. This treatment includes wearing shoes with a wide, tall toe box and level heel. A variety of toe sleeves to pad the toes are available commercially. Budin splints help reduce deformity, stabilize the MTP joint, and pad the metatarsal head. Surgical correction is indicated when conservative measures fail and the patient experiences significant pain and disability. In the neuropathic patient, surgical correction should be considered sooner if an ulcer has formed or is impending. When hammer toes are longstanding, the deformity transitions from being flexible to rigid, with the joints becoming arthritic and fixed. The surgical correction of rigid hammer toes is described elsewhere in this issue. When the deformity is still flexible, one can consider soft-tissue procedures to achieve correction. As with any soft-tissue balancing procedure, a thorough understanding of the deforming forces as described previously is essential to a successful outcome.

Isolated flexor tenotomies may improve mild and flexible flexion deformities at the PIP joint but do not address other factors in more complex deformities. Tamir and colleagues[12] showed that isolated percutaneous flexor tenotomies are effective to alleviate active ulcers or prevent ulcer formation in diabetic clawtoes. Jacobs and Vandeputte[6] showed isolated FDL z-lengthening and FDB tenotomy to be effective in the pediatric population. The mainstay of surgical treatment of the flexible hammer toe deformity is the FDL flexor to extensor transfer.[13] First described by Girdlestone[14] and Taylor[15] for neurogenic clawtoes, their original description has been modified over the years and adapted for correcting flexible hammer toe deformities. The flexor to extensor transfer is designed to relieve the flexion-deforming force on the IP joints

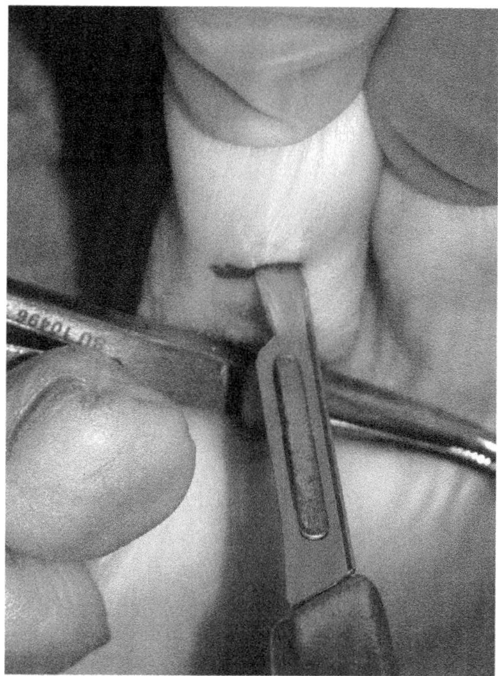

Fig. 4. Transverse incision made at the level of the distal plantar flexion crease to release the FDL.

while also reestablishing appropriate flexion at the MTP. Bayod and colleagues[16] demonstrated that the flexor to extensor transfer, although not as successful in reducing dorsal displacement of the proximal phalanx compared with PIP arthrodesis, is a more successful operation for reducing tensile and compressive stresses to the phalanges.

TECHNIQUE

To perform the flexor to extensor technique, the patient is first placed supine on the operating table. The authors' preference is to have the patient's heel centered on the edge of the operative table. After standard preparation and draping, the foot is exsanguinated with an Esmarch wrap. It is the authors' preference to avoid an ankle tourniquet in favor of a midcalf one to avoid trapping the tendons.

A small incision is made transversely on the plantar side at the proximal plantar flexion crease at the level of the PIP joint. Typically there is a small vein that requires cautery. Small retractors are placed, and the flexor tendon sheath is identified. The sheath is incised, and a small hemostat is inserted under both flexor tendons (**Fig. 3**). At this level the surgeon will see both slips of the FDB flanking the centrally located FDL tendon. The FDL is the larger, with a distinct median raphe. Pulling the tendon will result in flexion at the DIP joint, providing further clarification.

Next, through a small transverse "stab" incision made at the level of the distal plantar flexion crease (under the DIP joint), the FDL is percutaneously released off of the base of the distal phalanx using a #11 blade (**Fig. 4**). The FDL tendon is pulled through the proximal incision and split longitudinally along its median

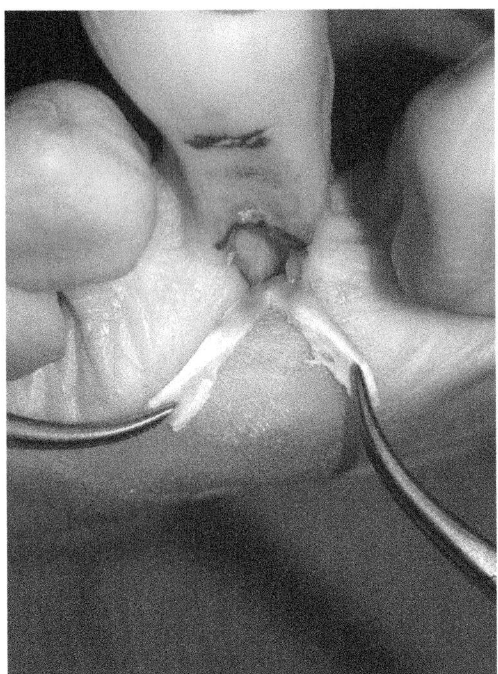

Fig. 5. Splitting the tendon along the median raphe to create two limbs.

raphe, creating a medial and lateral limb (**Fig. 5**). A dorsal longitudinal midline incision is made over the toe from the MTP to the PIP joint. A small curved hemostat is bluntly passed from dorsal to plantar both medially and laterally. Care must be taken to advance the hemostats against the bone so as not to entrap the neurovascular bundle when transferring the flexor limbs dorsally. Each end of the split FDL is grasped and passed dorsally and superficial to the extensor hood (**Fig. 6**). A knot is tied in the tendon loosely (**Fig. 7**).

Next, the toe is hyperflexed at the MTP joint and a Kirschner wire is driven antegrade from the MTP joint out the distal aspect of the toe. The toe is correctly positioned with approximately 20° of MTP plantarflexion, the wire is drilled retrograde into the metatarsal head, and the knotted FDL transfer is tied and finally secured to the extensor hood using 4-0 Vicryl suture.

The authors' preference is to release the Esmarch tourniquet at this time to look for adequate blood distal blood flow as demonstrated by capillary refill. If inadequate perfusion is noted, nitroglycerin paste is applied to the skin overlying the digital arteries both medially and laterally, and the toe is observed in the operating room. Adequate perfusion is usually restored in several minutes. If perfusion is not restored, the authors' preference is to then dangle the foot in sterile fashion off the operative table so as to break through any potential vasospasm of the artery. If perfusion is still not restored after several minutes, the toe can be repositioned to a more neutral position by gently bending the wire. The authors' preference is to not leave the operating theatre until perfusion is confirmed, although in the authors' experience, in most cases additional nitropaste and a heat lamp in the postoperative care unit have restored perfusion.

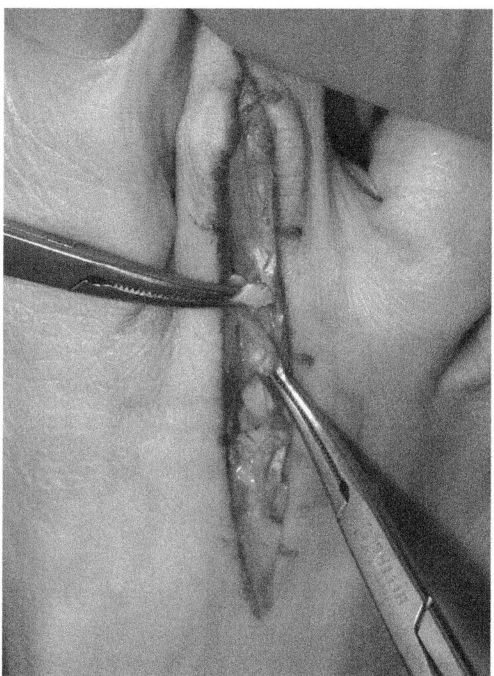

Fig. 6. Each end of the split FDL is passed dorsally and superficial to the extensor hood through the dorsal incision.

The pin is bent at the tip of the toe 100° dorsally and cut and capped. The skin is closed using 3-0 nylon suture in vertical mattress fashion. Often the authors use a chromic suture to place a simple interrupted suture plantarly. A sterile dressing is applied, and a postoperative shoe is placed.

Alternatively, Kuwada and colleagues[17,18] described a modification to the previously described fixation. This technique entails drilling a small pilot hole through the proximal phalanx, plantar to dorsal. The FDL, which does not need to be split in this procedure, is passed through the tunnel dorsally and secured to the extensor hood with sutures. Gazdag and colleagues,[19] however, reported no difference in outcomes using this technique versus more traditional techniques as described previously.[19] The authors do not perform an FDB transfer. Garcia-Gonzalez and colleagues[20] demonstrated in a finite-element simulation that FDB transfer results in a small but more uniform distribution of stress along the entire toe when compared with FDL transfer. Others have demonstrated that FDB transfer may be a viable alternative to FDL transfer.[21,22] Typically the plantar plate is not repaired, although Bouche and Heit[23] demonstrated that combined plantar plate repair with FDL transfer was effective in 18 cases for correction of chronic plantar plate tears with sagittal plane secondary joint instability and digital deformity.

Postoperatively, the patient is allowed to bear weight in a postoperative shoe. The sutures are removed at 2 weeks, and the pin is removed in the office at 3 to 4 weeks. The toe is then taped in correct alignment for 3 to 6 weeks. Range of motion of the toe is initiated at the 6-week mark, and the patient is transitioned

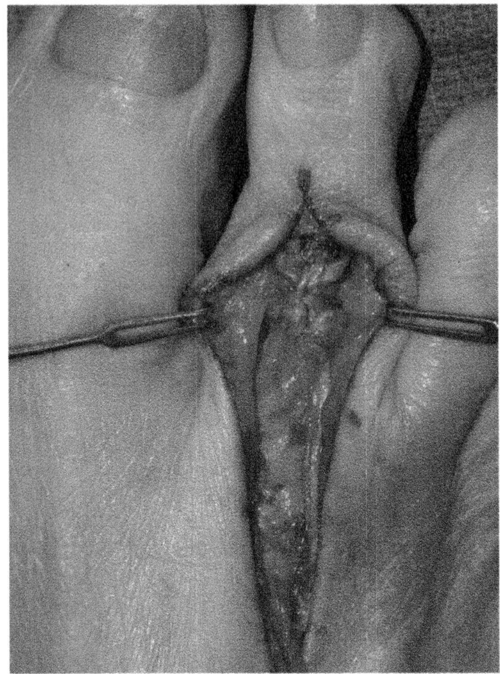

Fig. 7. The two limbs of the split tendon are tied in a knot dorsally and secured with suture.

into a regular shoe. Formal physical therapy is usually not required for isolated hammer toe repair.

COMPLICATIONS

Complications are uncommon but can range from infection, numbness, pin loosening, recurrent deformity, and incomplete correction to vascular injury and ischemia. If a pin is placed across the MTP joint, it can break.[24] Should a pin break occur, removal might require an MTP joint arthrotomy. Fracture of the phalanx, although rare, was described in a case report by Fishco and Roth.[25] Thompson and Deland[26] observed excellent postoperative pain relief but noted only 54% of those with a subluxated MTP joint had achieved complete correction at follow-up. It should be explained to patients preoperatively that they will lack normal motor control of the toe. Additionally, patients may experience generalized stiffness or "floating" of the toe.

Reported satisfaction rates are inconsistent, ranging from 51% to greater than 90%.[15,17,27–31]

SUMMARY

Flexor to extensor transfer is a useful means for the correction of a flexible hammer toe deformity. Although satisfaction rates have varied in the literature, this technique remains a useful tool in the surgeon's armamentarium to improve toe deformity, decrease pain, and aid in shoe wear.

REFERENCES

1. Coughlin MJ. Common causes of pain in the forefoot in adults. J Bone Joint Surg Br 2000;82(6):781–90.
2. Coughlin MJ. Lesser toe abnormalities. J Bone Joint Surg Am 2002;84:1446–69.
3. Coughlin MJ. Operative repair of the mallet toe deformity. Foot Ankle Int 1995;16(3): 109–16.
4. Coughlin MJ, Dorris J, Polk E. Operative repair of the fixed hammer toe deformity. Foot Ankle Int 2000;21(2):94–104.
5. Boyer A. A treatise on surgical diseases, and the operations suited to them, vols I-II [Stevens AH, Trans.]. New York: T & J Swords, 1815-16. p. 383–385.
6. Jacobs R, Vandeputte G. Flexor tendon lengthening for hammer toes and curly toes in paediatric patients. Acta Orthop Belg 2007;73(3):373–6.
7. Coughlin MJ, Thompson FM, The high price of high-fashion footwear. Instr Course Lect 1995;44:371–37.
8. Reece AT, Sonte MH, Young AB. Toe fusion using Kirschner wires. A study of of the postoperative infection rate and related problems. J R Coll Surg Edinb 1987;32(3): 157–9.
9. Scheck M. Etiology of acquired hammer toe deformity. Clin Orthop Relat Res 1977;123:63–9.
10. Fortin PT, Myerson MS. Second metatarsophalangeal joint instability. Foot Ankle Int 1995;16(5):306–13.
11. Haddad SL, Sabbagh RC, Resch S, et al. Results of flexor-to-extensor and extensor brevis tendon transfer for correction of the crossover second toe deformity. Foot Ankle Int 1999;20(12):781–8.
12. Tamir E, McLaren AM, Gadgil A, et al. Outpatient percutaneous flexor tenotomies for management of diabetic claw toe deformities with ulcers: a preliminary report. Can J Surg 2008;51(1):41–4.
13. Boyer ML, DeOrio JK. Transfer of the flexor digitorum longus for the correction of lesser-toe deformities. Foot Ankle Int 2007;28(4):422–30.
14. Girdlestone GR. Physiotherapy for hand and foot. Physiotherapy 1947;32:167–9.
15. Taylor RG. An operative procedure for the treatment of hammer-toe and claw-toe. J Bone Joint Surg Am 1940;22:607–9.
16. Bayod J, Losa-Iglesias M, Becerro de Bengoa-Vallejo R, et al.Advantages and drawbacks of proximal IP joint fusion versus flexor tendon transfer in the correction of hammer and claw toe deformity. A finite-element study. J Biomech Eng 2010;132(5): 051002.
17. Kuwada GT. A retrospective analysis of modification of the flexor tendon transfer for correction of hammer toe. J Foot Surg 1988;27(1):57–9.
18. Kuwada GT, Dockery GL. Modification of the flexor tendon transfer procedure for the correction of flexible hammer toes. J Foot Surg 1980;19(1):38–40.
19. Gazdag A, Cracchiolo A 3rd. Surgical treatment of patients with painful instability of the second metatarsophalangeal joint. Foot Ankle Int 1998;19(3):137–43.
20. Garcia-Gonzalez A, Bayod J, Prados-Frutos JC, et al. Finite-element simulation of flexor digitorum longus or flexor digitorum brevis tendon transfer for the treatment of claw toe deformity. J Biomech 2009;42(11):1697–704.
21. McCain LR. Transplantation of the flexor digitorum brevis in hammer toe surgery. J Am Podiatry Assoc 1958;48(6):233–5.
22. Beccero de Bengoa Vallejo R, Viejo Tirado F, Prados Frutos JC, et al. Transfer of the flexor digitorum brevis. J Am Podiatr Med Assoc 2008;98(1):27–35.

23. Bouche RT, Heit EJ. Combined plantar plate and hammertoe repair with flexor digitorum longus tendon transfer for chronic, severe sagittal plane instability of the lesser metatarsophalangeal joints: preliminary observations. J Foot Ankle Surg 2008; 47(2):125–37.
24. Zingas C, Katcherian DA, Wu KK. Kirschner wire breakage after surgery of the lesser toes. Foot Ankle Int 1995;16(8):504–9.
25. Fishco WD, Roth BJ. Digital fracture after a flexor tendon transfer for hammertoe repair: a case report. J Foot Ankle Surg 2010;49(2):179–81.
26. Thompson FM, Deland JT. Flexor tendon transfer for metatarsophalangeal instability of the second toe. Foot Ankle 1993;14(7):385–8.
27. Barbari SG, Brevig K. Correction of clawtoes by the Girdlestone-Taylor flexor-extensor transfer procedure. Foot Ankle 1984;5(2):67–73.
28. Daly PJ, Johnson KA. Treatment of painful subluxation or dislocation at the second and third metatarsophalangeal joints by partial proximal phalanx excision and subtotal webbing. Clin Orthop Relat Res 1992;(278):164–70.
29. Parrish TF. Dynamic correction of clawtoes. Orthop Clin North Am 1973;4(1):97–102.
30. Pyper JB. The flexor-extensor transplant operation for claw toes. J Bone Joint Surg Br 1958;40(3):527–33.
31. Taylor RG. The treatment of claw toes by multiple transfers of flexor into extensor tendons. J Bone Joint Surg Br 1951;33-B(4):539–42.

Metatarsalgia: Distal Metatarsal Osteotomies

Reinhard Schuh, MD[a,*], Hans Joerg Trnka, MD[b]

KEYWORDS

- Chevron osteotomy • Closing wedge osteotomy
- Metatarsalgia • Metatarsophalangeal joints • Weil osteotomy

Metatarsalgia is among the most common sources of pain in the human body. Some use the term broadly to refer to a number of painful conditions in the forefoot. However, metatarsalgia has been differentiated from other forefoot conditions and is defined as pain across the plantar forefoot beneath the second, third, and fourth metatarsal heads. The many causes of metatarsalgia can be categorized in 3 groups: (1) Local disease in the region (eg, interdigital neuroma), (2) altered forefoot biomechanics (clawtoe, hallux rigidus), and (3) systemic disease affecting the region (rheumatoid arthritis).[1]

For all causes, the first-line treatment is nonoperative therapy. This includes shoe modification (stiff sole, retrocapital metatarsal bar), custom foot orthoses with a metatarsal pad, and gastrosoleus stretching exercises. Additionally, corticosteroid injections as well as shaving of callosities can be carried out. However, if nonoperative treatment fails, operative options are considered.

PATHOBIOMECHANICS

To understand pathobiomechanic mechanisms causing metatarsalgia, the basic principles of the gait cycle have to be understood. The cycle is divided into two phases: Stance phase (60% of the normal gait cycle) and swing phase (40% of the normal cycle). The forefoot is in contact with the ground throughout approximately half of the gait cycle. In normal stance, the metatarsal heads all should rest evenly on the floor. The first, fourth, and fifth metatarsals are mobile in the sagittal plane. The second and third metatarsals are relatively fixed in position by rigid articulations with their corresponding cuneiforms.[1] During walking, the foot functions as a 3-rocker mechanism, providing physiologic balance between forward movement of the body and stability of the foot and leg during the stance phase.[2–4]

The heel represents the first rocker, beginning with heel strike during the first 10% of the gait cycle. Metatarsalgia that is present in this particular phase of gait is usually

The authors have nothing to disclose.

[a] Department of Orthopaedics, Vienna General Hospital, Medical University of Vienna, Waehringer Guertel 18-20, Vienna 1180, Austria
[b] Foot and Ankle Center Vienna, Alserstrasse 43/8D, Vienna 1080, Austria
* Corresponding author.
E-mail address: reinhard.schuh@meduniwien.ac.at

Foot Ankle Clin N Am 16 (2011) 583–595
doi:10.1016/j.fcl.2011.08.009
foot.theclinics.com

caused by congenital deformities, for example, cavus foot or tight gastrosoleus complex. A cavus foot has an abnormal increase in longitudinal arch, which places weight bearing on the heel and metatarsal heads, with little or no support from the lateral plantar midfoot. The toes commonly remain in extension at the metatarsophalangeal (MTP) joint with the greater flexion angles of the corresponding metatarsals. Weight-bearing pressure is concentrated under the metatarsal heads as a result of the abnormal foot position. Forefoot varus increases the amount of weight bearing on the lateral aspect of the foot and leads to increased pressures under the fifth metatarsal head. In similar manner, forefoot valgus increases pressure under first the metatarsal head.[1]

The ankle is the second rocker during the next 20% of gait. In this phase (flat foot), the entire foot contacts the ground. Forefoot overloading occurs in this phase if ankle range of motion is restricted and if the plantarflexion of the metatarsals is increased.[5] The pressure transfers rapidly toward the forefoot after heel strike. During toe off, pressure moves rapidly toward the digits, primarily to the great toe. The first ray (first metatarsal or great toe) participates in 50% of weight bearing, the lesser rays contribute the other 50% (**Fig. 1**).

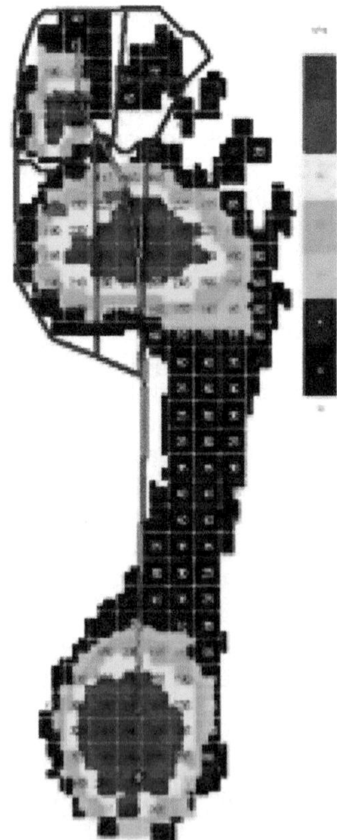

Fig. 1. Physiologic plantar pressure distribution during the stance phase of gait. During toe-off, the pressure moves rapidly to the great toe. This is shown by the deviation of the line that indicates the center of pressure in the forefoot area. The hallux is the major weight-bearing structure of the forefoot during stance phase of gait.

During the third rocker (toe off), only the forefoot is in contact with the ground and the MTP joints are dorsiflexed. Therefore, deformities of the MTP joints can produce metatarsalgia. Additionally, pathologic conditions on one metatarsal can cause overload of its neighbors. Hallux valgus alters first ray mechanics interrupting the windlass mechanism and weakening great toe flexion, which causes metatarsalgia (**Fig. 2**). Hallux rigidus, first ray hypermobility and iatrogenic weakening of the first MTP joint are common causes of metatarsalgia.[5]

CLINICAL EVALUATION

Evaluation of the patient starts with a careful history and physical examination.[6] A thorough patient history is taken and the foot is evaluated in weight-bearing and non–weight-bearing positions. History is focused on localizing pain, onset of symptoms, and alleviating or aggravating factors. The magnitude of deformity and the

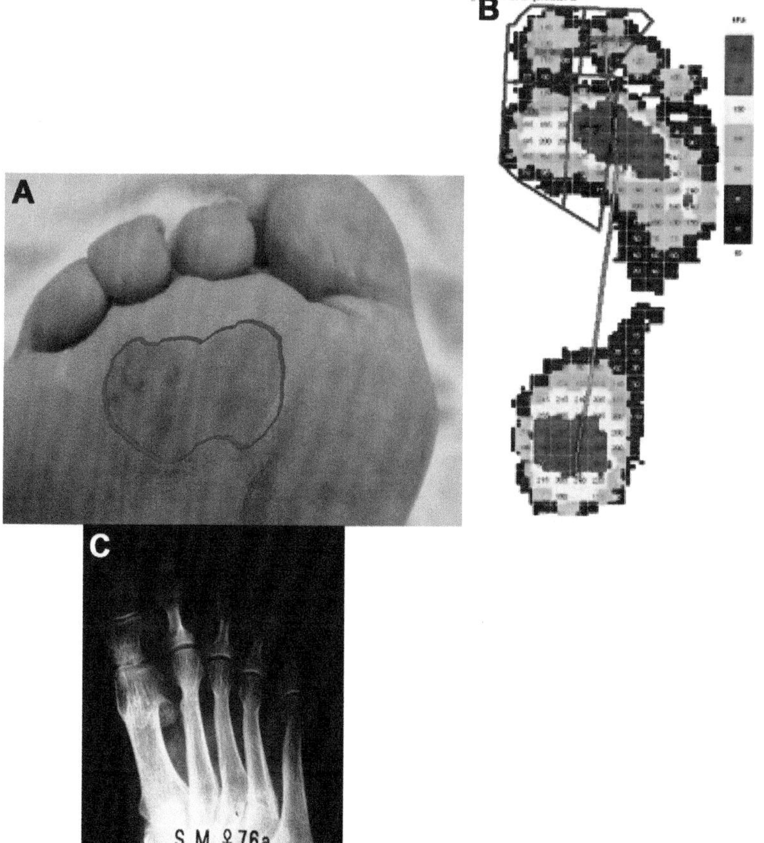

Fig. 2. (*A*) Foot of a patient with third rocker keratosis at the MTP 2 to 4 region owing to first ray insufficiency after Keller-Brandes resectional arthroplasty of the first MTP joint. (*B*) Plantar pressure analysis of the same patient. The pink and red areas indicate central overload. There is a lateralization of the center of pressure owing to first ray insufficiency and almost no weight bearing of the first ray. (*C*) Corresponding dorsoplantar x-ray.

effect of shoe wear on the foot are identified. It is important to note skin changes and deformities such as clawtoes, hammer toes, and hallux valgus, which can contribute to increased pressure under the metatarsal heads.

Assessing plantar calluses may give clues as to the pathology involved. Second rocker keratosis is strictly plantar under the metatarsal head. The foot should be evaluated for abnormal plantarflexion of the lesser metatarsals. Other causes of second rocker keratosis include gastrosoleus contracture and pes cavus. These keratoses do not show a tendency to extend distally toward the toes.

In contrast, third rocker keratosis is found more distal under the affected heads (see **Fig. 2**A). Each keratosis may be diffuse and span several heads. Keratosis associated with first ray insufficiency (ie, hallux valgus, hallux rigidus) exhibit third rocker features.[5]

After inspection, the foot is palpated and functional evaluation is performed. Palpation begins systematically, from the front to the rear. The goals of palpation are the assessment of topographic anatomy and recognition of any deviations. All bony prominences, anatomic regions, and metatarsals should be palpated. The plantar aspect of the foot along with each digit must be examined for the development of callosities and MTP alignment.[6] Each intermetatarsal web space is palpated to assess for tenderness of the interdigital nerves.[5]

Stability of the MTP joints in the sagittal and transversal plane must be tested. The examiner stabilizes the metatarsal neck in 1 hand and attempts to displace the base of the proximal phalanx with the other hand while holding the joint in the neutral position (toe Lachman test).

Hypermobility of the first ray and restricted dorsiflexion at the first MTP joint should be noted as well as hallux rigidus.[7] In addition, inversion and eversion range of motion of the hindfoot as well as medial columns stability should be evaluated.[5]

All muscles should be checked to assess strength and function. The Silfverskiöd method is used to evaluate for contracture of the gastrosoleus complex. Ankle dorsiflexion is tested with the knee in full extension and in 90° of flexion; the foot is maintained in an inverted position to avoid dorsiflexion movements at the midtarsal joints. Increased ankle dorsiflexion with the knee flexed indicates contracture of the gastrocnemius muscles.[5]

To provide a biomechanically objective investigation, dynamic plantar pressure distribution analysis can be performed. This reveals a reproducible image of plantar load distribution and may contribute to the therapeutic algorithm.

Radiographic Evaluation

Standard dorsoplantar and lateral weight-bearing radiographic views are obtained to evaluate the whole foot. The dorsoplantar view helps to identify MTP joint congruency, arthritis, and metatarsal length, as well as the degree of hindfoot deformity accompanying the forefoot deformity. There is typically a clear space of 2 to 3 mm between the metatarsal and adjacent phalanx. As the MTP hyperextends, the clear space diminishes and the phalanx subluxes dorsally over the metatarsal head. This is demonstrated on an anteroposterior radiograph as a diminished clear space and an overlapping adjacent bone.[8] If metatarsus primus varus is present, hallux valgus angle and intermetatarsal angle can be assessed as well on dorsoplantar views. In a radiographic study, Maestro and co-workers[9] introduced measures to assess forefoot geometry in detail on the dorsoplantar view. The lateral view can show collapse of the medial longitudinal arch and depict the magnitude of MTP joint dislocation to preoperatively gauge shortening.

Bone scans and magnetic resonance imaging can be helpful adjuncts in the inspection of neoplasm and infection, whereas computed tomographic scans can depict complex traumatic injuries. Neither is typically necessary in the management of metatarsalgia, however. Ultimately, imaging should support the clinical examinations and the decision for operative intervention.[6]

Preoperative Planning

Preoperative planning plays a crucial role in assessing the feasibility of an individual procedure and optimizing clinical outcomes. An accurate differential diagnosis, extensive understanding of disease pathophysiology, and knowledge of associated symptoms enables the surgeon to properly identify the lesions amendable for operative correction.

The 3-rocker assessment of gait helps to determine the necessary procedure. First rocker pathologies are usually caused by complex hindfoot deformities, and a simple distal metatarsal osteotomy is insufficient. In this situation, the underlying cause needs to be addressed, such as correction of the cavo varus deformity or an Achilles tendon lengthening. Second rocker gait pathologies are caused by decreased dorsiflexion of the ankle joint or plantarflexed metatarsals. This can be either corrected operatively to increase the ankle dorsiflexion or with a proximal metatarsal elevation osteotomy. Classical indications for distal metatarsal osteotomies are third rocker of gait pathologies like MTP subluxations or dislocations, crossover toe deformities, or relative overlength of the lesser metatarsal, whether congenital or acquired. One must be thorough in evaluating the entire lower extremity because global foot deformities can influence outcomes when addressing forefoot pathology.[6]

Lauf and Weinraub[10] used lateral x-rays to estimate the symptomatic metatarsal declination angle (β) and the clinically determined amount of metatarsal head elevation (Δh). A trigonometric formula, $\Delta h = X (\text{sine } \beta)$, where X is the unknown amount of bone that needs to be resected to yield the desired elevation, can theoretically be used intraoperatively to measure shortening.[10] Although this is certainly an important theoretical consideration, it is cumbersome for usage in clinical work. In the operating room, the authors usually determine the necessary amount of shortening on the preoperative standing radiographs. For a single shortening, the adjacent lesser metatarsal head is palpated and the proximal translation of the osteotomy is performed to equalize this length difference. The standard thickness of wedge resection is usually 3 mm (1 mm bone slice plus 1 mm each for the saw blade thickness).

Operative Techniques

The goal of the operation is to improve plantar pressure distribution within the forefoot after failure of nonoperative treatment. Lesser metatarsal osteotomy is an effective and well-accepted method for the management of metatarsalgia. The main purpose of these osteotomies is to decrease prominence of the symptomatic metatarsal head. This can be done by dorsiflexing the metatarsal head, shortening the metatarsal head, or some combination thereof. Accurate correction is important because insufficient shortening or elevation leads to recurrent metatarsalgia, whereas overzealous correction results in transfer lesions to the adjacent metatarsals. Depending on the underlying pathology, the surgeon must decide whether it is necessary to address metatarsalgia with lesser metatarsal osteotomy only or if additional procedures, such as Achilles tendon lengthening, flexor-to-extensor tendon transfer or repair of the plantar plate are necessary.[1,5]

All techniques can be performed under a regional ankle block with an Esmarch bandage as a tourniquet if needed. The senior author prefers forefoot surgery without tourniquet, which helps to limit postoperative swelling and edema.

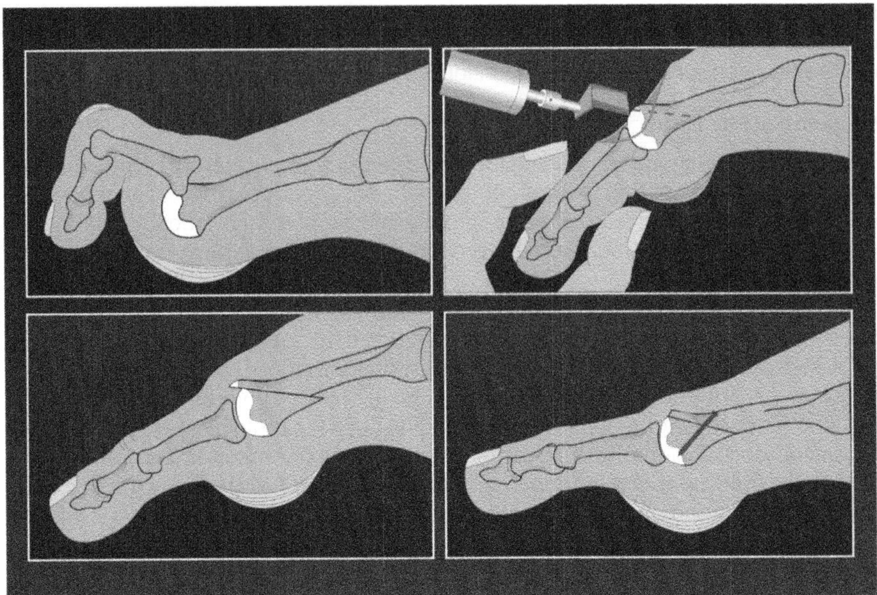

Fig. 3. Major steps of the Weil osteotomy in case of a dislocated MTP joint.

Distal Oblique Metatarsal Osteotomy (Weil Osteotomy)

The Weil osteotomy was first described by in 1985 for the treatment of central metatarsalgia. In 1992, it was introduced in France by Barouk.[11,12] The goal of a Weil osteotomy is to achieve adequate proximal translation of the metatarsal head in relation to the callus and to more evenly distribute pressure underneath the forefoot with adequate metatarsal–ground contact during third rocker. It is an intra-articular osteotomy that achieves longitudinal decompression through shortening.[5] A schematic drawing of the principles of this osteotomy is presented in **Fig. 3**.

A dorsal, 3-cm, longitudinal incision is made over the metatarsal for a single osteotomy and over the web space for adjacent osteotomies. In most cases, a *z*-type lengthening of the short and long extensor tendons is performed. After identifying the metatarsal head and neck, the joint capsule is incised. A laminar spreader is now inserted to expose the metatarsal. The laminar spreader is the instrument of choice since when using Hohmann retractors the saw blade will blocked by the retractors. The collateral ligaments of the MTP joint are cut, the dislocation of the MTP joint is partly reduced, and the toe is flexed to give optimal exposure of the metatarsal head. According to the original technique by Barouck, the plane of the osteotomy is parallel to the ground as if the foot was bearing weight.

Cadaveric studies have shown that, in clinical use, this is almost impossible and it has led to recurrent metatarsalgia. With our technique, we routinely resect a bony wedge of 3 to 4 mm to avoid plantar displacement with the proximal translation. After removal of the free bony slice, the plantar mobile fragment is then grasped with a pointed clamp and shifted proximally to achieve the requisite amount of shortening. After checking the positioning with the image intensifier, the two fragments are secured with a special titanium snap-off screw or a solid cortical lag screw. We recommend the 2-mm twist-off screw (Wright Medical, Arlington, TN, USA) rather than standard cortical lag screws or Kirschner wires for fixation of the Weil osteotomy. Most of

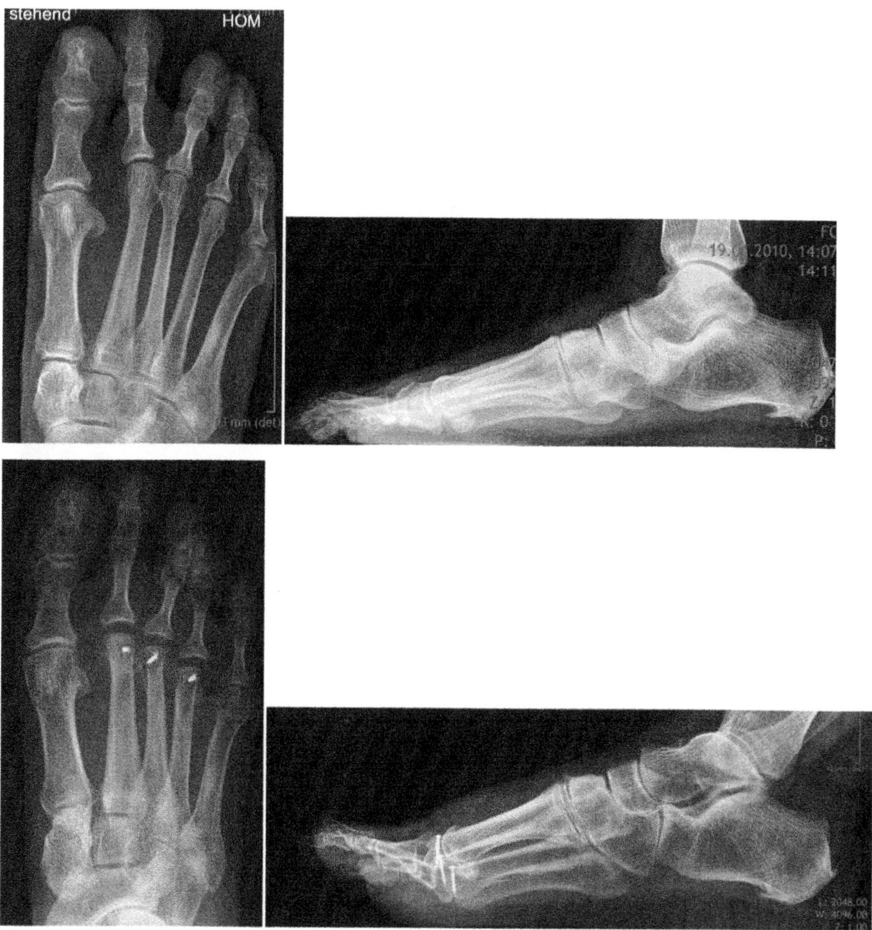

Fig. 4. Preoperative and postoperative dorsoplantar and lateral radiographs of a patient with third rocker metatarsalgia owing to a relatively short first ray and crossover toe deformity of the second toe. The patient underwent Weil osteotomy of the second, third, and fourth metatarsal heads. The clear space of the MTP joint is increased postoperatively, which indicates decompression of the joints.

the available minifragment screws require predrilling, which may displace the plantar fragment. The twist-off screw is used without predrilling and offers acceptable fixation in most cases. The resulting dorsal protuberance on the metatarsal head is then resected.[13] Weight bearing in a postoperative shoe is allowed immediately after surgery.[14]

Fig. 4 shows the dorsoplantar and lateral x-ray of a patient with third rocker metatarsalgia owing to a relatively short first ray and cross over toe deformity of the second toe. The patient underwent Weil osteotomy of the second, third, and fourth metatarsal heads.

Good to excellent results have been reported in 70% to 100% of patients treated with conventional Weil osteotomy.[13,15–18] Postoperative complications include MTP joint stiffness, floating-toe deformity, local second rocker metatarsalgia resulting from plantar shift of the lesser metatarsal head, transfer metatarsalgia caused by extensive

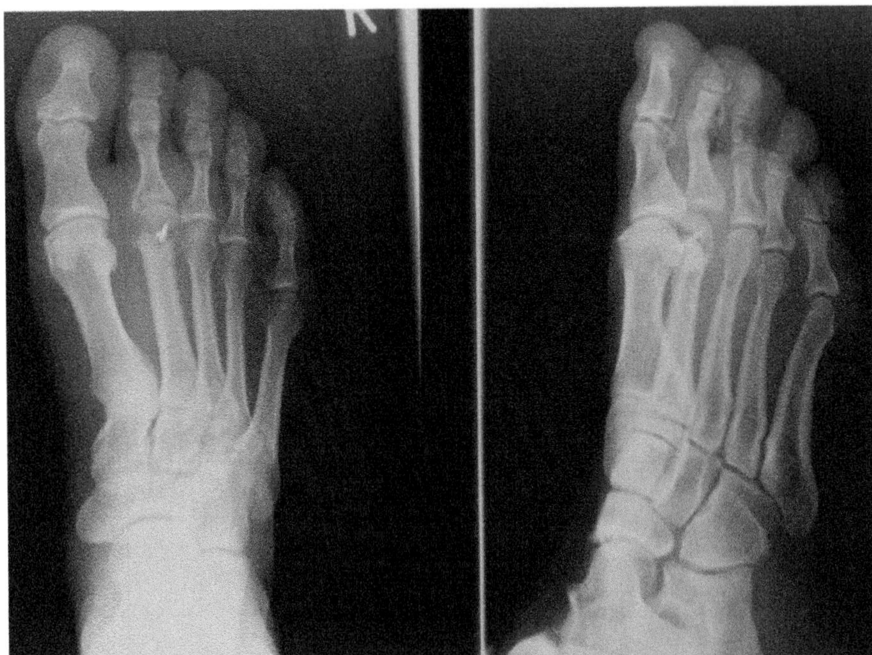

Fig. 5. Radiograph 6 months after Weil osteotomy of the second metatarsal. Nonunion occurred.

shortening, nonunion (**Fig. 5**), superficial wound healing problems, and complex regional pain syndrome.[5] The floating toe and MTP joint stiffness are the most common postoperative complications. One reason is the dorsal approach to the joint capsule, which may lead to postoperative contracture and cocking up of the toe. Another reason may be insufficiency of the plantar plate, which can lead to dorsal subluxation of the MTP joint and a floating toe. Our solution is lengthening of the extensor tendons and, if possible, a reconstruction of the plantar plate by transosseous sutures of the distal plantar plate through the base of the proximal phalanx. In some obvious cases of dorsal dislocation intraoperatively, we pass a 1.4-mm K-wire from the toe through the metatarsal head across the osteotomy into the proximal metatarsal shaft. Postoperative taping of the toes may also help to avoid subsequent cocking up of the toe.

In a cadaveric study, our group investigated biomechanical changes of the interosseous muscles after performing conventional Weil osteotomy in 4 different angles in relation to the longitudinal axis of the metatarsal (25°–40°). We found that the tendons of the interosseous muscles moved dorsally in relation to the MTP joint owing to depression of the plantar fragment of the metatarsal. This leads to loss of their flexion moment on the MTP joint. Therefore, the pull of the extensor leads to dorsiflexion of the toe and the interosseous muscles act as a synergist for dorsiflexion of the MTP joint. The amount of depression ranged from 3.0 to 4.6 mm, depending on the angle of the osteotomy. We concluded that the investigated biomechanical changes may explain the commonly seen dorsiflexion contracture after Weil osteotomy. Based on the results of this cadaveric study, the following modifications were recommended: (1) Lengthening of the extensor tendon(s), (2) making the osteotomy plane as parallel as possible to the ground surface, (3) adding a flexor to extensor transfer, and (4) inserting a Kirschner wire from the tip of the toe across the MTP joint and the osteotomy into the MTP joint (in a position of 5° of plantar flexion). The Kirschner wire prevents dorsiflexion during soft tissue healing, but intensive physiotherapy after 4 weeks is necessary toe prevent stiffness of the joint.[19] Because flexor to extensor tendon transfer leads to bulky dorsal soft tissue and increases the likelihood of wound healing problems, we have abandoned this procedure.

To avoid complications associated with the traditional Weil osteotomy, Maceira and colleagues[20] introduced a 3-step modification of the Weil osteotomy. This modification aims to recreate a more anatomic metatarsal, with preservation of the relative length and position of the interossei musculature in relation to the center of rotation of the MTP joint. In addition, the shape and integrity of the cartilage of the metatarsal head are not altered. The direction of shortening of the conventional Weil osteotomy runs mostly parallel to the plantar aspect of the foot, whereas in the triple Weil osteotomy it is coaxial to the bone. Espinosa and co-workers[5] reported low rates of MTP joint stiffness and floating toe deformity with the 3-step technique. Potential complications include osteonecrosis of the metatarsal head, infection, synostosis, plantar migration of the hardware, and neurovascular impairment.[5]

Benichou performed another extra-articular modification of the conventional Weil osteotomy by doing a step cut keeping the plantar cortex of the distal fragment.[12]

If the MTP joint is not affected (no subluxation or dislocation) in case of crossover toe deformity or isolated overlength of the metatarsal, the authors perform the Weil osteotomy in an extra-articular fashion by starting the cut at the metadiaphyseal junction of the distal metatarsal region.

Vandeputte and associates[17] evaluated plantar pressure distribution in addition to clinical results after Weil osteotomy. The investigations have been performed pre- and postoperatively. They noted a reduction of plantar pressure under the operated metatarsal head in all but 1 patient. The mean decrease was 1.0 kg/cm^2. The decrease in pressure corresponded to a good clinical result and showed a correlation between pressure reduction and patient outcome.[17]

Recently, minimally invasive modifications of Weil osteotomy have been introduced.[21] However, there is no evaluation of such methods in the peer-reviewed literature to date.

Author's Preferred Technique for the Modified Weil Osteotomy

The senior author prefers a modified Weil osteotomy in the majority of cases. The key step in this modification that differs from the originally described technique includes the removal of a slice of bone at the osteotomy site. Theoretically, this improves the plantar pressure relief in the forefoot region; however, this has not been definitively proven biomechanically.

The surgery is performed using a regional ankle block for anesthesia, and supplement with intravenous or oral sedation. An Esmarch-tourniquet may be used to obtain a bloodless field. A 3-cm, longitudinal incision is made dorsal over the metatarsal for a single osteotomy, over the web space for a double osteotomy. A small amount of soft tissue dissection is done to identify the extensor tendons, which is lengthened in a *Z*-fashion. A transverse or longitudinal capsulotomy of the MTP joint is made to identify the junction of the head and neck. The metatarsal head is exposed with a laminar spreader. Care is taken not to strip the plantar soft tissue attachments to aid in stabilizing the osteotomy and maintain vascularity to the head.[22] The dislocation of the MTP joint is partly reduced and the toe is flexed plantar to give optimal exposure of the metatarsal head. After that, a 1- to 2-mm bony slice

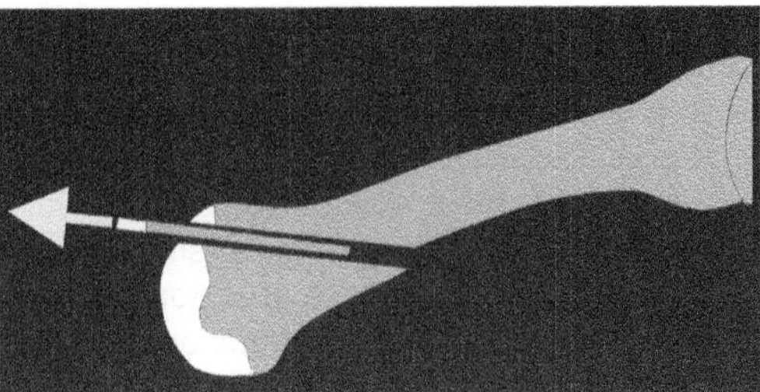

Fig. 6. Removal of the bony slice to achieve elevation of the metatarsal head.

extraction is desired to lift the dorsal fragment because the axis of motion of the MTP joint has changed with plantar flexion of the metatarsal head (**Figs. 6** and **7**). In this abnormal case, the interosseous muscle act as dorsiflexor rather than plantarflexor and result in a contracted subluxated MTP joint.[19] Using an oscillating saw, the osteotomy aims from the dorsal portion of the metatarsal head proximally. The second osteotomy through both cortices is 2 mm under the dorsal cut. The bony slice can now be easily removed.

The plantar mobile fragment is then grasped with a pointed reduction clamp and is shifted proximally to achieve the requisite amount of shortening that was measured preoperatively on the dorsoplantar radiographs. The plane of the osteotomy has to be as parallel to the ground surface as possible. The osteotomy was secured with a special 2 mm titanium "Twist off screw" (Wright Medical). We have abandoned the K-wires for fixation of the Weil osteotomy and recommend the "twist-off" screw for fixation of the osteotomy. Most of the available minifragment screws require predrilling, which may dislocate the plantar fragment. The so-called twist-off screw is used without predrilling. The resulting dorsal protuberance over the metatarsal head remnant was removed with a rongeur. Finally the overlying *Z*-lengthened extensor tendon is repaired and the skin sutured.

Although the classical Weil osteotomy is an intra-articular procedure indicated for sagittal plane MTP dislocation, horizontal plane pathologies like crossover toe

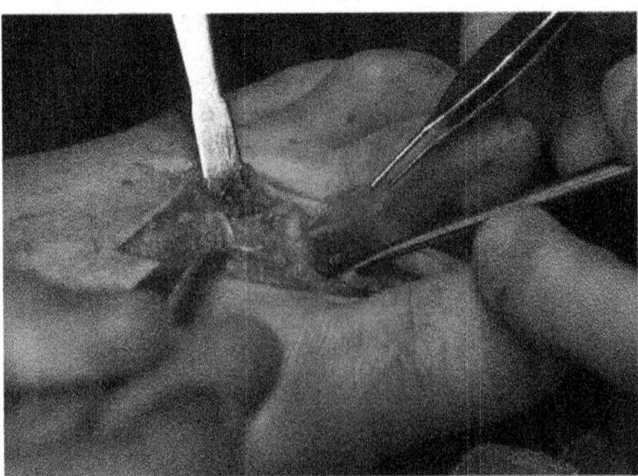

Fig. 7. Intraoperative situation after double osteotomy and removal of the bony slice in a patient who underwent modified Weil osteotomy of the second metatarsal for the treatment of metatarsalgia caused by subluxation of the second MTP joint (third rocker of gait metatarsalgia).

deformities might benefit from maintaining the dorsal joint. In these cases, an extra-articular Weil osteotomy with wedge resection is performed. The difference to the classic Weil osteotomy is that this osteotomy is performed proximal to the joint capsule. Adequate elevation can be achieved by resection of a bony slice. Shortening and decompression of the MTP joint pressure can be achieved by pushing the plantar fragment proximally, with standard 2.0-mm cortical screws used for fixation.

Distal Metatarsal V (Closing Wedge) Osteotomy

Leventen and Pearson first described this type of osteotomy as a modification of the method described by Wolf.[23–25] It represents a *V*-shaped osteotomy with a plantar apex. It is carried out in the metadiaphyseal junction of the metatarsal. Wolf originally determined the diaphysis of the metatarsal as location of the osteotomy and recommended to perform it at 1 metatarsal at each stage.[25] To avoid transfer lesions, Leventen and Pearson followed a set protocol. If the hyperkeratosis was located under the second metatarsal head only, the second and third metatarsal heads were addressed surgically. If the hyperkeratosis was under the fourth metatarsal head, osteotomies of the third and fourth metatarsal were performed. If hyperkeratosis was present underneath the third metatarsal head, osteotomies of the second to fourth metatarsal were carried out.

After the MTP joint is approached in usual manner, a V-shaped trough is made in the dorsal three fourths of the metatarsal neck using a rongeur. This trough is 5 mm at its widest point. The osteotomy is closed using manual pressure. No fixation is used. Patients are encouraged to weight bear to keep the osteotomy closed 24 hours after the procedure.

Leventen and Pearson reported in 1987 in 21 feet a decrease of subjective pain score from 7.7 to 1.3. Five patients continued to have metatarsalgia, one of them worsened postoperatively. Sixteen patients were completely satisfied, two were satisfied, and three were dissatisfied.[23] We have no personal experience performing this technique, and it seems to be more of historical interest.

Chevron Osteotomy

Kitaoka and Platzer[26] described a distal chevron osteotomy for the treatment of metatarsalgia. The apex of the cut was centered at the metadiaphyseal junction of the metatarsal. The limbs of the osteotomy were at 45° directed proximally and the cut made vertically relative to the metatarsal. The distal fragment was displaced dorsally approximately 2 to 3 mm and manually impacted. The authors believed the osteotomy was stable, but used internal fixation with a short threaded Kirschner wire.

In their series, they reported pain relief in 15 of a total of 19 patients. Two patients required revision surgery owing to severe residual pain. Three patients suffered transfer metatarsalgia. The mean amount of shortening with this osteotomy was 2.6 mm. With the dorsally directed force of weight bearing in line with the osteotomy, however, excess dorsal displacement is possible without internal fixation. When performing this osteotomy, it is wise to use internal fixation. If fixation is not performed, there may be increased risk of transfer metatarsalgia.

SUMMARY

Metatarsalgia is a common pathologic entity. It refers to pain at the MTP joints. Pain in the foot unrelated to the MTP joints (such as Morton's neuroma) must be distinguished from those disorders, which lead to abnormal pressure distribution, reactive calluses, and pain.

Initial treatment options for metatarsalgia include modifications of shoe wear, metatarsal pads, and custom-made orthoses. If conservative treatment fails, operative reconstructive procedures in terms of metatarsal osteotomies should be considered. Lesser metatarsal osteotomy is an effective and well-accepted method for the management of metatarsalgia. The main purpose of these osteotomies is to decrease prominence of the symptomatic metatarsal head. The distal metatarsal oblique osteotomy (Weil osteotomy) with its modification represents the best evaluated distal metatarsal osteotomy in terms of outcome studies and biomechanical analysis. The role of the Weil osteotomy in metatarsalgia owing to a subluxed or dislocated MTP joint is to bring the metatarsal head proximal to the callus and to provide axial decompression of the toe to correct the deformity contributing to metatarsalgia.

REFERENCES

1. Feibel JB, Tisdel CL, Donley BG. Lesser metatarsal osteotomies. A biomechanical approach to metatarsalgia. Foot Ankle Clin 2001;6:473–89.
2. Perry J. Gait analysis: Normal and pathologic function. Thorofare (NJ): Slack Inc.; 1992.
3. Daniels T, Thomas R. Etiology and biomechanics of ankle arthritis. Foot Ankle Clin 2008;13(3):341–52.
4. Bober T, Dziuba A, Kobel-Buys K, et al. Gait characteristics following Achilles tendon elongation: the foot rocker perspective. Acta Bioeng Biomech 2008;10:37–42.
5. Espinosa N, Brodsky JW, Maceira E. Metatarsalgia. J Am Acad Orthop Surg 2010;18:474–85.
6. Hamilton KD, Anderson JG, Bohay DR. Current concepts in metatarsal osteotomies: a remedy for metatarsalgia. Techniques in Foot & Ankle Surgery 2009;8:77–84.
7. Grebing BR, Coughlin MJ. The effect of ankle position on the exam for first ray mobility. Foot Ankle Int 2004;25:467–75.
8. Davis H, Mann R. Principles of the physical examination of the foot and ankle. In: Coughlin M, Mann R, Saltzmann C, editors. Surgery of the foot and ankle. Philadelphia: Mosby, Elsevier; 2007. p. 45–70.
9. Maestro M, Besse JL, Ragusa M, et al. Forefoot morphotype study and planning method for forefoot osteotomy. Foot Ankle Clin 2003;8:695–710.
10. Lauf E, Weinraub GM. Asymmetric "V" osteotomy: a predictable surgical approach for chronic central metatarsalgia. J Foot Ankle Surg 1996;35:550–9.
11. Viladot A. To Weil or not to Weil. Abstractbook of the 8th International Congress of the European Foot and Ankle Society. Geneva, 2010.
12. Maestro M. Weil: YES! Why? Abstractbook of the 8th International Congress of the European Foot and Ankle Society. Geneva, 2010.
13. Hofstaetter SG, Hofstaetter JG, Petroutsas JA, et al. The Weil osteotomy: a seven-year follow-up. J Bone Joint Surg Br 2005;87:1507–11.
14. Schuh R, Trnka HJ, Sabo A, et al. Biomechanics of postoperative shoes: plantar pressure distribution, wearing characteristics and design criteria: a preliminary study. Arch Orthop Trauma Surg 2010;131:197–203.
15. Trnka HJ, Gebhard C, Muhlbauer M, et al. The Weil osteotomy for treatment of dislocated lesser metatarsophalangeal joints: good outcome in 21 patients with 42 osteotomies. Acta Orthop Scand 2002;73:190–4.
16. Hart R, Janecek M, Bucek P. The Weil osteotomy in metatarsalgia. Z Orthop Ihre Grenzgeb 2003;141:590–4.
17. Vandeputte G, Dereymaeker G, Steenwerckx A, et al. The Weil osteotomy of the lesser metatarsals: a clinical and pedobarographic follow-up study. Foot Ankle Int 2000;21:370–4.

18. Jarde O, Hussenot D, Vimont E, et al. Weil's cervicocapital osteotomy for median metatarsalgia: report of 70 cases. Acta Orthop Belg 2001;67:139–48.
19. Trnka HJ, Nyska M, Parks B, et al. Dorsiflexion contracture after the Weil osteotomy: results of cadaver study and three-dimensional analysis. Foot Ankle Int 2001;22:47–50.
20. Maceira E, Farinas F, Tena J, et al. Analysis of metatarsophalangeal stiffness following Weil osteotomies. Rev Med Cir Pie 1998;12:35–40.
21. De Prado M. Principles of percutaneous and MIS. Abstractbook of the 8th International Congress of the European Foot and Ankle Society. Geneva, 2010.
22. Sammarco G, Scioli MW. Metatarsal osteotomy using a double threaded compression screw. Foot Ankle Int 1989;10:129–39.
23. Wolf M. Metatarsal osteotomy for the relief of painful metatarsal callosities. J Bone Joint Surg Am 1973;55:1760–2.
24. Kitaoka H, Platzer GL. Chevron osteotomy of lesser metatarsals for intractable plantar callosities. J Bone Joint Surg Br 1998;80:516–8.
25. Petersen WJ, Lankes JM, Paulsen F, et al. The arterial supply of the lesser metatarsal heads: a vascular injection study in human cadavers. Foot Ankle Int 2002;23:491–5.
26. Leventen E, Pearson SW. Distal metatarsal osteotomy for intractable plantar keratosis. Foot Ankle Int 1987;10:274-51.

Metatarsalgia: Proximal Metatarsal Osteotomies

Christopher J. Pearce, FRCS (Tr&Orth), MFSEM (UK)[a,*],
James D. Calder, MD, FRCS (Tr&Orth), FFSEM (UK)[b]

KEYWORDS

• Metatarsalgia • Metatarsal • Osteotomy • Treatment
• Complications

Metatarsalgia is a generic term, derived from the Greek, to describe pain in the forefoot. It is generally accepted to mean pain that is felt around the plantar aspects of the lesser metatarsal heads but it does not give any specific clue as to the cause of the pain or how best to treat it.[1] The various causes of metatarsalgia can be broadly classified as local, biomechanical, or systemic abnormalities,[2] and a careful history and examination of the patient is required to ascertain exactly which part of the forefoot is involved and to elucidate which contributory factors exist. Metatarsalgia is a common complaint that is frequently seen in patients attending a foot and ankle clinic. Patients often describe the symptoms by saying that they feel like they are walking on "marbles" or with a "rolled-up sock" under a foot.[3] The exact incidence varies depending on the underlying condition but in one postal survey study of patients with rheumatoid arthritis, 93.5% of respondents reported having experienced foot pain in the past and 35.4% reported current foot pain at the time of the study, with the majority of this pain felt in the forefoot.[4] Women have a higher incidence of metatarsalgia than men, which is often attributed to the wearing of shoes with high heels and narrow toe boxes, resulting in substantially greater pressure being borne by the metatarsal heads.[2]

Some authors prefer to categorize metatarsalgia according to primary and secondary causes, with iatrogenic often added as a third category.[5–7] Primary metatarsalgia occurs due to an underlying anatomic abnormality in the foot or ankle resulting in increased pressure under the metatarsal heads and pain. Examples of primary causes of metatarsalgia include congenitally short or long metatarsals relative to each other (the most common being a relatively long second metatarsal as in the Morton type foot[8,9]), first ray instability, forefoot equinus, hind foot equinus including tight

The authors have nothing to disclose.
[a] Department of Orthopaedics, Jurong Healthcare (Alexandra Hospital), 378 Alexandra Road, Singapore 159964
[b] Department of Orthopaedics, Chelsea and Westminster Hospital, 369 Fulham Road, London, SW10 9NH, UK
* Corresponding author.
E-mail address: chris.pearce@doctors.net.uk

Foot Ankle Clin N Am 16 (2011) 597–608
doi:10.1016/j.fcl.2011.08.007
foot.theclinics.com

gastrocnemius or Achilles tendon,[10] and anatomic abnormalities in the shape of the metatarsal heads themselves. Secondary causes of metatarsalgia include inflammatory arthropathies, most notably rheumatoid arthritis, trauma, hallux rigidus, neuropathic pain as in Morton metatarsalgia,[11] and osteonecrosis (Freiberg infraction). Iatrogenic metatarsalgia occurs as a result of failed forefoot surgery resulting in actual or apparent length discrepancies in the metatarsals or discrepancies in the metatarsal head heights.

The mainstay of treatment in metatarsalgia is nonoperative. Having said this, there is little written about the effectiveness of nonoperative treatments in metatarsalgia.[5] Clearly, the risk of complications occurring with nonoperative measures is very low, and the use of such treatments does not preclude surgical intervention at a later date. Nonoperative interventions include the use of calf-stretching programs, which can be supervised by a physical therapist, in cases of Achilles or gastrocnemius tightness. The use of orthotics such as a metatarsal bar or dome insoles and shoe modifications such as rocker-bottom soles may be attempted to off-load pressure from the affected forefoot. Painful plantar callosities may be pared down to provide temporary relief of associated pain, but treatment of the underlying cause of the callosity is required for a permanent solution. Injections of local anesthetic or steroid in selected cases, for example, into the metatarsophalangeal (MTP) joint in cases of synovitis or, under ultrasound guidance into a Morton neuroma, may be helpful both diagnostically and potentially therapeutically[11,12] but one needs to be mindful of the possible, albeit rare, complications with these including fat pad atrophy, lipodystrophy, and infection.[5,11,13] Metatarsalgia caused by a structural abnormality may prove resistant to conservative therapy, however, and operative intervention may be necessary.[14]

SURGICAL TREATMENT

Surgical treatment of metatarsalgia is indicated when conservative measures have failed to improve the patient's symptoms. Surgical planning requires a sound knowledge of what biomechanical parameters need to be corrected and what associated conditions need to be addressed. The overall aim of surgical intervention is to restore a normal pressure distribution to the forefoot while minimizing complications. Sometimes this may be achieved by procedures away from the forefoot itself such as gastrocnemius recession to reduce plantar pressure in patients with an isolated gastrocnemius contracture, which remains refractory to a stretching program.[15] This procedure has been shown to produce an enhanced range of ankle motion and self-reported function while not inducing any detrimental effects to plantar flexion strength.[16] In other cases, where the metatarsalgia and abnormal plantar loading of the lesser metatarsal heads is due to shortening or instability of the first ray, addressing the first ray abnormality may be all that is required. In a recent study by Lee and coworkers, 40 patients with painful plantar callosities under the lesser metatarsal heads underwent correction of their hallux valgus alone with a proximal chevron osteotomy. Among these patients, 92.5% experienced complete pain relief from their metatarsalgia, with 80% having no residual callosity at a mean follow-up of 26 months.[17] Where there is gross instability at the first tarsometatarsal joint (TMTJ), a Lapidus procedure (TMTJ arthrodesis) may be utilized. Where the first ray dysfunction is due to metatarsus primus varus with less obvious hypermobility at the first TMTJ, either a Lapidus fusion or the various first metatarsal osteotomies may be used alone or in combination with lesser metatarsal procedures.[14,17–19] It is often preferable to achieve some plantar displacement of the first metatarsal head to create the correct biomechanical environment and offload the lesser metatarsal heads.[20,21]

There are several lesser metatarsal osteotomies described, and these may be performed at the distal, middle, or proximal portions of the metatarsal. Proximal osteotomies in general are more powerful than distal ones in that a small correction at the base of the bone will translate into a large correction at the head due to the long lever arm. This may be an advantage where considerable correction is required as well as having the advantages of an extra-articular osteotomy. Avascular necrosis (AVN) after lesser metatarsal surgery is a recognised complication,[22,23] and another possible advantage of a proximal osteotomy over a distal one is that the blood supply to the lesser metatarsal head is less likely to be affected. Work by Petersen and colleagues[24] showed that the metatarsal heads are supplied by dorsal and plantar metatarsal arteries that are branches of the dorsalis pedis and posterior tibial arteries, respectively. They typically form an anastomosis around the metatarsal heads that may be disrupted by surgery in this area. However, the incidence of AVN after lesser metatarsal osteotomy generally is very low and is certainly less frequently reported than that after first metatarsal osteotomy.[25,26]

However, although more powerful, proximal osteotomies tend to be less forgiving if not carefully positioned and can lead to subsequent imbalance and transfer metatarsalgia. There is also concern that the long lever arm produced by a proximal osteotomy could impair bone healing[5] by increasing strain at the osteotomy site. Therefore, careful attention must be paid to not only the creation and displacement of the osteotomy but also to its fixation in order to prevent complications.

Distal metatarsal osteotomies are the subject of another article by Hans Joerg Trnka elsewhere in this issue and therefore are not covered in any detail here.

Whether the osteotomy is to be performed proximally or distally, the surgeon needs to decide whether the aim of the procedure is to elevate or shorten the metatarsal head or both. Clinical examination and radiographic evaluation together are used to make these decisions. It may be apparent that the problem is primarily one of a short first ray, especially in cases of iatrogenic shortening secondary to previous hallux valgus surgery. The patient's second toe will often be longer than the first and palpation will reveal the relatively short position of the first metatarsal head with respect to the second, and sometimes even the third. **Fig. 1** is an AP weight-bearing radiograph of a 65-year-old woman who presented with severe metatarsalgia 15 years after a Wilson's osteotomy for hallux valgus. Note the significant shortening of the first metatarsal. In this case, because the second and third MTP joints were dislocated, the big toe remains longer than the second on inspection but palpation of the plantar aspects of the metatarsal heads, along with the radiographs, reveals the cause of her metatarsalgia. She also had significant tightness in her gastrocnemius, which compounded the problem of lesser metatarsal head overload. In this case, shortening of the second and third metatarsals by sliding osteotomies along with gastrocnemius recession were recommended.

Alternatively, on inspection there does not appear to be an abnormality in the relative lengths of the metatarsals but the head of one or more may be elevated or depressed with respect to the others on palpation. There will often be a callosity over the more plantarly displaced head. **Fig. 2** reveals before and after computed tomography (CT) imaging of such a case in a running athlete who presented with pain and callus formation under the third metatarsal. The third metatarsal head was relatively plantar to the others preoperatively, and an elevating osteotomy relieved her symptoms.

In general it is desirable to maintain or restore the harmonious metatarsal cascade described by Maestro and colleagues[8] to ensure that there is correct and even ground contact for each metatarsal head and to limit the risk of producing transfer lesions.[5,27,28] It may therefore be necessary to shorten or elevate an asymptomatic ray

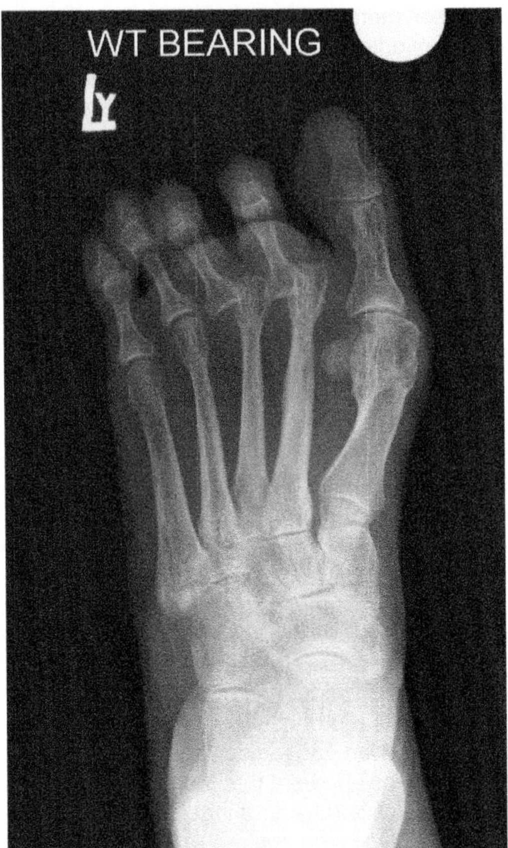

Fig. 1. Metatarsalgia with dislocation of second and third MTPs after iatrogenic shortening of the first metatarsal with a Wilson osteotomy. Note also the hypertrophic changes in the second metatarsal as a result of the transfer of load from the first to the second metatarsal.

to maintain the cascade. For example, when operating on a symptomatic second metatarsal leads to the third metatarsal head becoming the most prominent, the currently asymptomatic third may have to be operated on to prevent it from becoming symptomatic.

Proximal Lesser Metatarsal Osteotomies

Step-cut osteotomy

The step-cut metatarsal osteotomy (**Fig. 3**) was originally described by Giannestras[29,30] with the aim of shortening the symptomatic metatarsal. In his original paper, the osteotomy was created by making a series of drill holes and then completing the cut with an osteotome. Each limb of the step cut was 0.5 inch wide and the metatarsal was thus shortened by 0.5 inch. At that time, the osteotomy was held together with a catgut suture. In his series of 40 patients, 10% developed a transfer lesion while 37 of 40 were rated as having good to excellent results. This was a very demanding procedure, however, and some of the osteotomies mentioned in the sections that follow were evolutions of the theme, in pursuit of a technically simpler procedure.

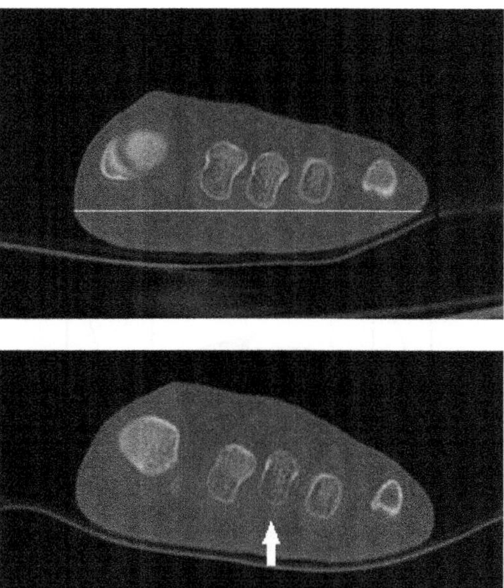

Fig. 2. CT images at the level of the metatarsal heads before and after elevating proximal osteotomy (BRT) of the third metatarsal.

Oblique diaphyseal metatarsal osteotomy

The oblique diaphyseal sliding osteotomy procedure was originally described by Mann and Coughlin.[31] After a dorsal approach the metatarsal shaft is exposed. Before the osteotomy is cut, a transverse mark is made in the metatarsal at the midportion of the osteotomy so that as the osteotomy site is displaced, the surgeon can measure

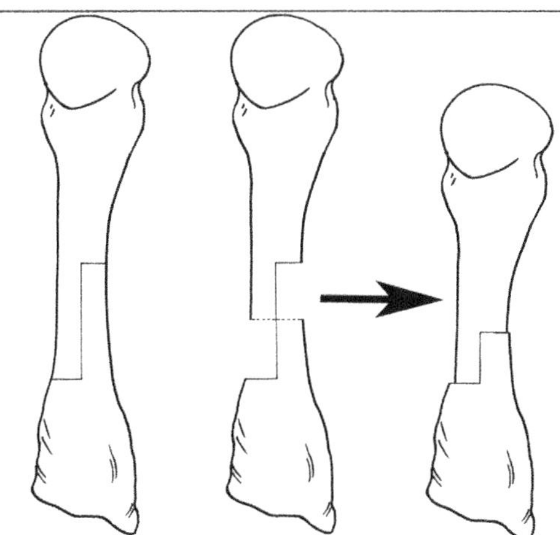

Fig. 3. The step-cut osteotomy. Each limb of the osteotomy was 0.5 inch long, resulting in overall metatarsal shortening of 0.5 inch.

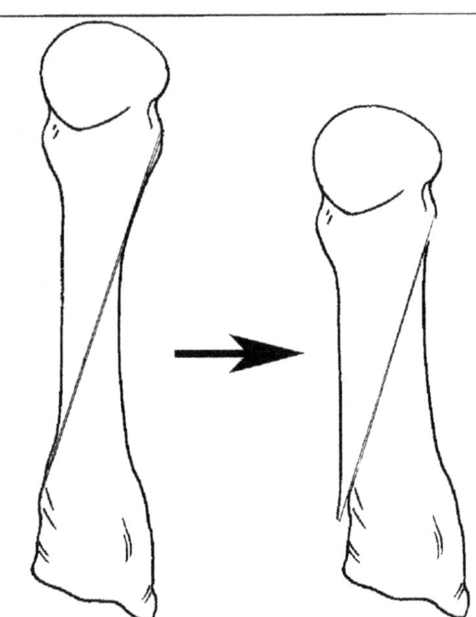

Fig. 4. The oblique diaphyseal sliding osteotomy as described by described by Mann and Coughlin.[31]

precisely how much shortening is being achieved. It is recommended that the deep transverse metatarsal ligament be sectioned if more than 5 to 6 mm of shortening is required. With a thin oscillating saw blade, an oblique osteotomy is made as long as possible in the metatarsal shaft (**Fig. 4**). Kennedy and Deland[32] pointed out the intraoperative flexibility of a slightly modified version of this procedure whereby the cut is made slightly off the midline of the metatarsal diaphysis to allow access for temporary pinning and final fixation. The position is checked both clinically and radiographically while held with clamps and, where necessary, adjusted before final fixation. In their series, 31 of 32 patients had relief of plantar pain with a mean time to radiographic union of 10 weeks (range, 8–15 weeks). Complications included one patient with ipsilateral toe numbness, three with a dorsiflexion contracture of the toe, and one callosity developed over the proximal interphalangeal joint after progressive plantar flexion of the proximal interphalangeal joint and dorsiflexion at the MTP joint. Despite these minor complications, no patient had any functional impairment. There were no non-unions but healing rates were noted to be slower than those reported for the Weil osteotomy.[32]

Slovenkai and coworkers[33] compared the biomechanical characteristics of two methods of fixation of oblique osteotomies in a cadaveric study. Although they stated their aim was to determine the best way of fixating metatarsal shaft fractures, the osteotomy that they produced was the same as the oblique osteotomy described in the preceding text. They found that the stiffness of the construct was significantly greater with a single lag screw than with crossed Kirschener wires.

Segmental osteotomy

Proximal segmental osteotomy (**Fig. 5**) without internal fixation, involving just a simple resection of a cylindrical segment of bone, approximately 0.5 cm long, was reported

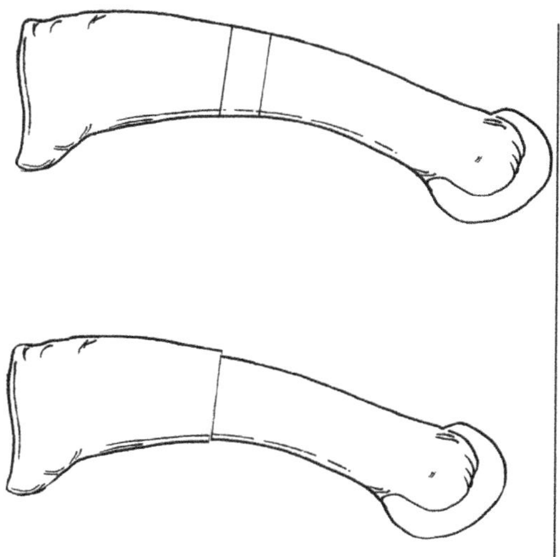

Fig. 5. The segmental osteotomy. Union rates are vastly improved when the osteotomy is fixed as described by Galluch and coworkers.[14]

by Spence and colleagues in 1990.[34] Good to excellent subjective results were reported at a mean of 6 years follow-up in 89% of these patients. Transfer lesions occurred in 18% of the feet and recurrent plantar keratoses developed in 7%. However, despite the high levels of patient satisfaction, other surgeons held an unfavorable opinion of this procedure because of the 76% non-union rate.

In 2007, Galluch and coworkers[14] reported the results of a retrospective series of lesser metatarsal midshaft, segmental osteotomy with open reduction and internal fixation. The operative technique that they describe[14,35] consists of a dorsal longitudinal incision centred over the metatarsal to the approximate length of the diaphysis. The metatarsal diaphysis is then exposed by blunt dissection and area only slightly larger than the size of a quarter tubular plate is exposed subperiosteally. A segment of metatarsal diaphysis for resection is marked with an oscillating saw and the two distal screw holes are drilled, tapped, and measured before the osteotomy is performed. The distal cut is made first, followed by the proximal cut, and saline is used to irrigate during the creation of the osteotomy to limit any thermal necrosis of the bone. The four-hole plate is pre-bent to approximately 5° in the middle, to allow compression of the plantar cortex, and is centered over the osteotomy. The distal aspect of the plate is secured by filling the two predrilled holes, and the two proximal screws are placed in compression mode. Autogenous local bone graft, obtained from drill reamings and the resected section of metatarsal, is packed around the metatarsal osteotomy. Postoperatively, a splint and then a cast, non-weight-bearing, is used for 2 months. Clinical outcomes were not reported in this paper because the majority of patients had concomitant surgery to other parts of the foot, which would have confounded the results. With the careful attention to surgical detail they described, 125 of their 126 osteotomies united (99.2%) which is comparable to that of the Weil osteotomy.[36] Another positive aspect of this technique is that it allows precise control over the metatarsal length, and the amount of bone to be resected can be tailored to the individual. A disadvantage when compared to, for example, the Weil osteotomy is the restriction on weight bearing that is required postoperatively.

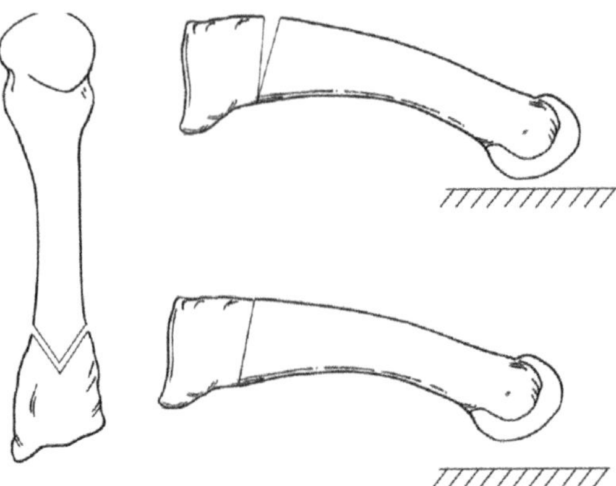

Fig. 6. The proximal V osteotomy demonstrating the elevation of the metatarsal head that it produces.

Proximal metatarsal V osteotomy

A dorsal proximal metatarsal V osteotomy was originally described by Sclamberg and Lorenz in 1983.[37] The V-shaped cut is made in the metatarsal with an oscillating saw with the apex facing toward the base of the metatarsal and at a 60° angle to the metatarsal shaft. The plantar cortex is left intact. A second V-shaped cut is then made 3 to 4 mm distally, converging toward the plantar cortex where the first cut ended. Downward pressure is then exerted over the metatarsal head until the plantar cortex cracks, the V-shaped wedge is removed, and then upward pressure applied to the plantar aspect of the metatarsal head to close the osteotomy and relieve the excess plantar pressure (**Fig. 6**). No fixation of the bone is undertaken in this technique. The original paper included 41 osteotomies. In all patients, relief of symptoms was achieved, plantar callosities were resolved, and no significant complications were reported.

BRT osteotomy

The BRT osteotomy was devised in 2000 by Barouk, Rippstein, and Toullec for the treatment of metatarsalgia and pes cavus deformities as well as failed previous forefoot surgery.[38] The surgical technique for what they describe as the *metatarsal oblique basal osteotomy (BRT)* is a long and as horizontal as possible cut in the proximal metaphysis with a thin oscillating saw blade. The cut starts distally on the dorsal surface and progresses proximally to the plantar surface, which is kept intact. A second cut is then made very close to the first, with the amount to be removed assessed by plantar palpation and under the metatarsal head to ascertain how much elevation is required (**Fig. 7**). The osteotomy is then fixed with a compression screw across the gap. It should be remembered that this osteotomy does not allow for shortening of the metatarsal; it is purely an elevation osteotomy. Also, as previously mentioned, often only a very small amount of bone needs to be removed because the osteotomy is a very powerful one, being so close to the base of the metatarsal. There are no published results of this technique in the English-language literature.

Authors' Preferred Approach

With a combination of a careful history and examination, it is usually possible to determine the likely primary cause for metatarsalgia. If the problem is one of length

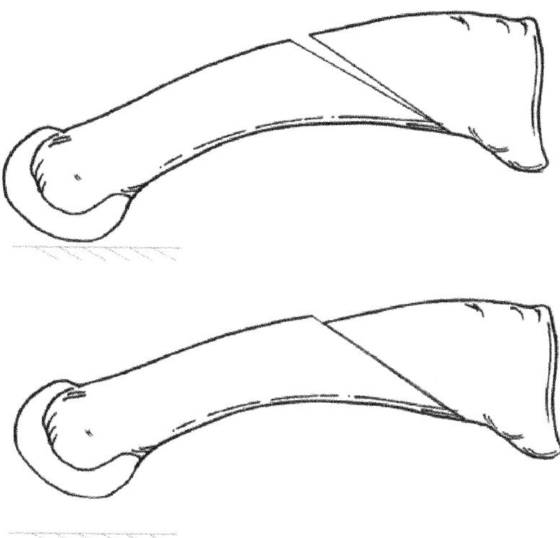

Fig. 7. The BRT osteotomy demonstrating the elevation of the metatarsal head that it produces. It is recommended that the osteotomy be fixated with a compression screw.

discrepancy (see **Fig. 1**), standard weight-bearing AP, oblique, and lateral radiographs are sufficient to confirm the diagnosis and plan surgery in terms of a shortening osteotomy. A shortening oblique sliding osteotomy rather than a pure elevating osteotomy is the preferred option in such cases. When there is a discrepancy in the relative heights of the metatarsal heads, further imaging in the form of a sesamoid or metatarsal head view radiograph (**Fig. 8**) or a CT scan can be useful to confirm the clinical suspicion and plan an elevating osteotomy. We use a BRT osteotomy fixed with a Barouk screw in these cases. We fix all of our osteotomies to mitigate against the risk of non-union.

Complications

Non-union

One of the main concerns regarding proximal metatarsal osteotomies is the risk of non-union. The long lever arm and the fact that diaphyseal osteotomies generally heal

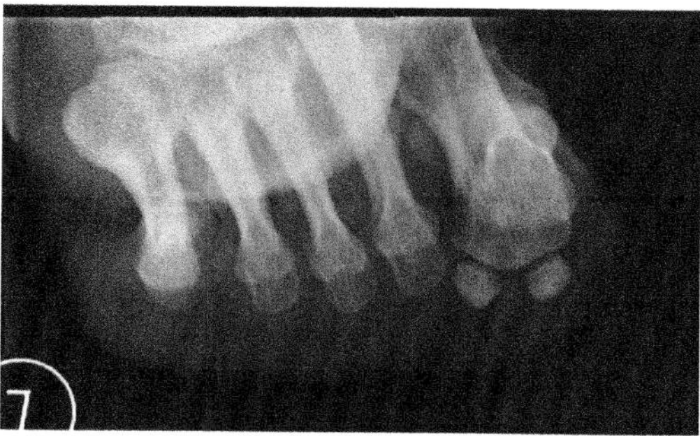

Fig. 8. Preoperative metatarsal head view showing excessive plantar displacement of the 3rd metatarsal head (from the same patient as in **Fig. 2**).

less well than metaphyseal osteotomies contribute to this complication. Up to 76% non-union rates have been described,[34] which is obviously unacceptably high in modern practice. The best way to avoid non-union appears to be by solid internal fixation, in which the non-union rate drops to around 1%.[14] Protected or non-weight-bearing for up to 6 weeks postoperatively may also be necessary when performing a diaphyseal as opposed to a distal metaphyseal osteotomy.

Transfer metatarsalgia

Transfer metatarsalgia is a potential complication of any osteotomy. Assuming that the osteotomy unites and remains in the position that it was fixed, the occurrence of transfer metatarsalgia is most likely due to an error in surgical planning or execution rather than a problem with the osteotomy itself. This complication can be avoided by maintaining the metatarsal cascade, which may involve surgery to several or sometimes all of the lesser metatarsals.

Cock-up toe deformity (floating toe)

Cock toe deformity theoretically should be less common with proximal osteotomies than with distal ones because they are extra-articular procedures. The only series of proximal osteotomies to mention this specifically was that of Kennedy and colleagues,[32] who reported a 10% incidence. This compares favorably to recent reports of up to 36% with the Weil osteotomy.[39] It is important that patients passively plantarflex operated lesser toes at the MTP joint after lesser metatarsal osteotomies in the postoperative period to try to stretch out the developing scar tissue and thus prevent this complication.

SUMMARY

Metatarsalgia is a blanket term to describe pain in the forefoot that may have many different etiologies and contributory factors. A careful history, examination, and appropriate imaging are required to make an accurate diagnosis and treat the patient appropriately. Metatarsalgia is a common condition and is more common in women. Many nonsurgical treatments can be implemented as a first line but if these fail then surgery may be undertaken. There are several different lesser metatarsal osteotomies described with little published evidence to recommend one over another, leaving the decision as to which one to use largely to surgeon choice. The surgeon, however, must decide, by using a combination of clinical examination and imaging, whether the desired effect of the osteotomy is to shorten or elevate the metatarsal head or both. Whichever method is employed it is important to maintain or restore the metatarsal cascade to keep even pressure under the lesser metatarsal heads and prevent transfer lesions. Proximal osteotomies are more powerful than distal ones but often that can mean that they are more technically demanding. Many early descriptions of osteotomy techniques did not include any fixation but the results in terms of union and relief of symptoms as well as the prevention of transfer pain appear to be better with fixation. More research is required comparing the different osteotomy techniques to ascertain which can most reliably resolve patients' symptoms with the lowest complication rate.

ACKNOWLEDGMENTS

The authors thank Yuki Maruko and Dr Sarah LaPorte for their help in producing the figures in this article.

REFERENCES

1. Coughlin MJ. Common causes of pain in the forefoot in adults. J Bone Joint Surg Br 2000;82(6):781–90.
2. Feibel JB, Tisdel CL, Donley BG. Lesser metatarsal osteotomies. A biomechanical approach to metatarsalgia. Foot Ankle Clin 2001;6(3):473–89.
3. Barouk P, Bohay DR, Trnka HJ, et al. Lesser metatarsal surgery. Foot Ankle Spec 3(6):356–60.
4. Otter SJ, Lucas K, Springett K, et al. Foot pain in rheumatoid arthritis prevalence, risk factors and management: an epidemiological study. Clin Rheumatol 2010; 29(3):255–71.
5. Espinosa N, Brodsky JW, Maceira E. Metatarsalgia. J Am Acad Orthop Surg 2010; 18(8):474–85.
6. Espinosa N, Maceira E, Myerson MS. Current concept review: metatarsalgia. Foot Ankle Int 2008;29(8):871–9.
7. Scranton PE, Jr. Metatarsalgia: a clinical review of diagnosis and management. Foot Ankle. 1981;1(4):229–34.
8. Maestro M, Besse JL, Ragusa M, Berthonnaud E. Forefoot morphotype study and planning method for forefoot osteotomy. Foot Ankle Clin 2003;8(4):695–710.
9. Rodgers MM, Cavanagh PR. Pressure distribution in Morton's foot structure. Med Sci Sports Exerc 1989;21(1):23–28.
10. DiGiovanni CW, Kuo R, Tejwani N, et al. Isolated gastrocnemius tightness. J Bone Joint Surg Am 2002;84-A(6):962–70.
11. Hassouna H, Singh D. Morton's metatarsalgia: pathogenesis, aetiology and current management. Acta Orthop Belg 2005;71(6):646–55.
12. Markovic M, Crichton K, Read JW, et al. Effectiveness of ultrasound-guided corticosteroid injection in the treatment of Morton's neuroma. Foot Ankle Int 2008;29(5): 483–7.
13. Kumar N, Newman RJ. Complications of intra- and peri-articular steroid injections. Br J Gen Pract 1999;49(443):465–6.
14. Galluch DB, Bohay DR, Anderson JG. Midshaft metatarsal segmental osteotomy with open reduction and internal fixation. Foot Ankle Int 2007;28(2):169–74.
15. Maskill JD, Bohay DR, Anderson JG. Gastrocnemius recession to treat isolated foot pain. Foot Ankle Int 2010;31(1):19–23.
16. Chimera NJ, Castro M, Manal K. Function and strength following gastrocnemius recession for isolated gastrocnemius contracture. Foot Ankle Int 2010;31(5):377–84.
17. Lee KB, Park JK, Park YH, et al. Prognosis of painful plantar callosity after hallux valgus correction without lesser metatarsal osteotomy. Foot Ankle Int 2009;30(11): 1048–52.
18. Coughlin MJ, Jones CP. Hallux valgus and first ray mobility. A prospective study. J Bone Joint Surg Am 2007;89(9):1887–98.
19. Coughlin MJ, Jones CP, Viladot R, et al. Hallux valgus and first ray mobility: a cadaveric study. Foot Ankle Int 2004;25(8):537–44.
20. Barouk LS. Scarf osteotomy for hallux valgus correction. Local anatomy, surgical technique, and combination with other forefoot procedures. Foot Ankle Clin 2000; 5(3):525–58.
21. Pearce CJ, Sexton SA, Sakellariou A. The triplanar chevron osteotomy. Foot Ankle Surg 2008;14(3):158–60.
22. Bayliss NC, Klenerman L. Avascular necrosis of lesser metatarsal heads following forefoot surgery. Foot Ankle 1989;10(3):124–8.

23. Bellacosa RA, Pollak RA. Complications of lesser metatarsal surgery. Clin Podiatr Med Surg 1991;8(2):383–97.
24. Petersen WJ, Lankes JM, Paulsen F, Hassenpflug J. The arterial supply of the lesser metatarsal heads: a vascular injection study in human cadavers. Foot Ankle Int 2002;23(6):491–5.
25. Green MA, Dorris MF, Baessler TP, et al. Avascular necrosis following distal Chevron osteotomy of the first metatarsal. J Foot Ankle Surg 1993;32(6):617–22.
26. Jones KJ, Feiwell LA, Freedman EL, Cracchiolo A 3rd. The effect of chevron osteotomy with lateral capsular release on the blood supply to the first metatarsal head. J Bone Joint Surg Am 1995;77(2):197–204.
27. Kitaoka HB, Patzer GL. Chevron osteotomy of lesser metatarsals for intractable plantar callosities. J Bone Joint Surg Br 1998;80(3):516–8.
28. Pontious J, Lane GD, Moritz JC, Martin W. Lesser metatarsal V-osteotomy for chronic intractable plantar keratosis. Retrospective analysis of 40 procedures. J Am Podiatr Med Assoc 1998;88(7):323–31.
29. Giannestras NJ. Shortening of the metatarsal shaft for the correction of plantar keratosis. Clin Orthop 1954;4:225–31.
30. Giannestras NJ. Shortening of the metatarsal shaft in the treatment of plantar keratosis; an end-result study. J Bone Joint Surg Am 1958;40–A(1):61–71.
31. Mann RA, Coughlin MJ. Intractable plantar keratosis. In: Mann RA. Coughlin MJ, editors. Video textbook of foot and ankle surgery, vol. 1. St. Louis (MO): Medical Video Productions; 1991.
32. Kennedy JG, Deland JT. Resolution of metatarsalgia following oblique osteotomy. Clin Orthop Relat Res 2006;453:309–13.
33. Slovenkai MP, Linehan D, McGrady L, et al. Comparison of two fixation methods of oblique lesser metatarsal osteotomies: a biomechanical study. Foot Ankle Int 1995; 16(7):437–9.
34. Spence KF, O'Connell SJ, Kenzora JE. Proximal metatarsal segmental resection: a treatment for intractable plantar keratoses. Orthopedics 1990;13(7):741–7.
35. Hamilton K, Holthusen S, Bohay DR, Anderson JG. Midshaft metatarsal segmental osteotomy with plate fixation. Oper Tech Orthop 2008;18:231–8.
36. Trnka HJ, Muhlbauer M, Zettl R, et al. Comparison of the results of the Weil and Helal osteotomies for the treatment of metatarsalgia secondary to dislocation of the lesser metatarsophalangeal joints. Foot Ankle Int 1999;20(2):72–9.
37. Sclamberg EL, Lorenz MA. A dorsal wedge V osteotomy for painful plantar callosities. Foot Ankle 1983;4(1):30–2.
38. Toullec E, Barouk LS, Rippstein P. Ostéotomie de relèvement basal Métatarsien BRT. Chirurgie de l'avant Pied Cahiers d'enseignement de la SOFCOT Coordination B. 2eme édition. Paris: Valtin et T. Leemrijse Elsevier; 2005. p. 142–8.
39. Highlander P, Vonherbulis E, Gonzalez A, et al. Complications of the Weil osteotomy. Foot Ankle Spec 2011;4(3):165–70.

The Crossover Toe and Valgus Toe Deformity

James Sferra, MD*, Steven Arndt, MD

KEYWORDS

• Crossover toe • Deformity • Pain • Treatment • Valgus toe

Because of its position next to the hallux, relative length of the second metatarsal, and limited motion at the second tarsometatarsal joint, pain, inflammation, and subluxation are common problems of the second metatarsophalangeal (MTP) joint. Crossover toe typically occurs when the second toe deviates medially and dorsally over the hallux, leaving an increased space between the second and third toes (**Fig. 1**). It also is common to see the second toe deviate laterally into a valgus deformity, often owing to a hallux valgus deformity and pressure from the great toe.

These deformities often begin with slight pain, likely owing to synovitis of the second MTP joint. This can be detected by localized pain and swelling at the second MTP. A positive drawer test of the second MTP may be elicited.[1] In the case of a crossover toe, the early pain and swelling may be followed by an increase in the space between the second and third toes (splaying) or a slight medial deviation of the second toe. As the deformity progresses, the capsuloligamentous structures, specifically the fibular collateral ligament, get stretched or torn on the lateral aspect of the MTP joint and the medial collateral ligament contracts, causing a deformity in the axial plane (**Fig. 2**). The plantar plate also attenuates on the lateral side and this fosters deformity in the sagittal plane. Global instability about the second MTP occurs with extension and medial deviation of the second toe, causing a crossover toe deformity. A grading system for second MTP joint subluxation (**Table 1**) has been developed that shows the progression and initial stages of MTP joint subluxation, crossover toe deformity, and ultimately frank dislocation of the MTP.[2]

ETIOLOGY

Many causes have been postulated to cause a crossover toe deformity. A marked hallux valgus deformity can crowd the second toe causing it to subluxate dorsomedially (**Fig. 3**). Hallux rigidus has also been associated with a second crossover toe deformity. Neuromuscular, congenital, and inflammatory arthritides can all cause crossover toe deformity. However, ill-fitting shoe wear combined

Cleveland Clinic Main Campus, Mail Code A40, 9500 Euclid Avenue, Cleveland, OH 44195, USA
* Corresponding author.
E-mail address: SFERRAJ@ccf.org

Foot Ankle Clin N Am 16 (2011) 609–620
doi:10.1016/j.fcl.2011.09.001
foot.theclinics.com
1083-7515/11/$ – see front matter

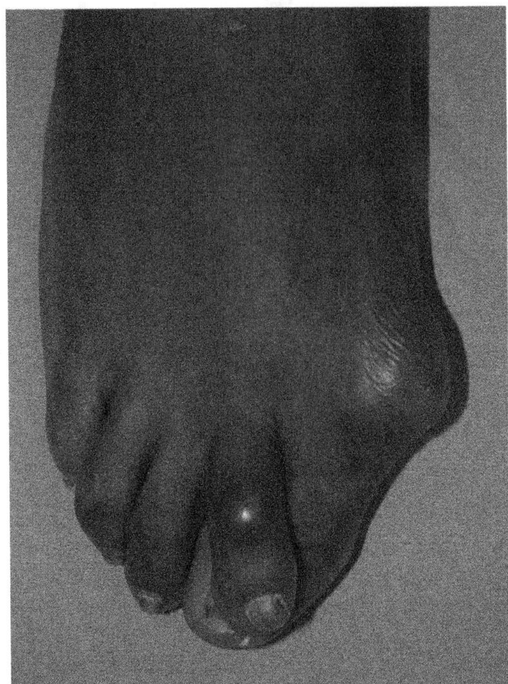

Fig. 1. Clinical image of crossover deformity of second toe.

with the aging process are the most likely causes. Certainly, with age, the incidence of developing a crossover toe increases. Anatomic abnormalities have also been implicated in crossover toe deformity. An elongated second ray (Morton foot) combined with repetitive stresses at the second MTP joint can create a reactive synovitis.[1] Further, repetitive injury to the plantar plate caused by buckling of the long second toe and chronic extension of the MTP attenuate the plantar plate, leading to extension deformity at the MTP. Anomalous muscles have also been speculated to cause this deformity. Hatch and Burns[3] described an accessory medial head of the extensor digitorum brevis (EDB) and noted its appearance in 4 out of 7 cadaveric specimens. They theorized that ability of the EDB to dorsiflex and adduct the second toe could contribute to a crossover toe deformity. Impingement from the third toe has also been implicated in crossover toe deformity. A traumatic episode can lead to a crossover toe deformity as well, after a dorsiflexion injury to the second MTP joint that tears the plantar plate and capsule.

CLINICAL PRESENTATION

Second crossover toe deformities most commonly occur in women over 50 years of age. High-heeled fashion shoe wear is also a common historical finding in these patients. Although traumatic events have been described as a cause, this deformity most commonly occurs as a chronic problem slowly developing over several months to years. There exists a relatively high association between problems of the hallux—both hallux valgus and hallux rigidus—and crossover

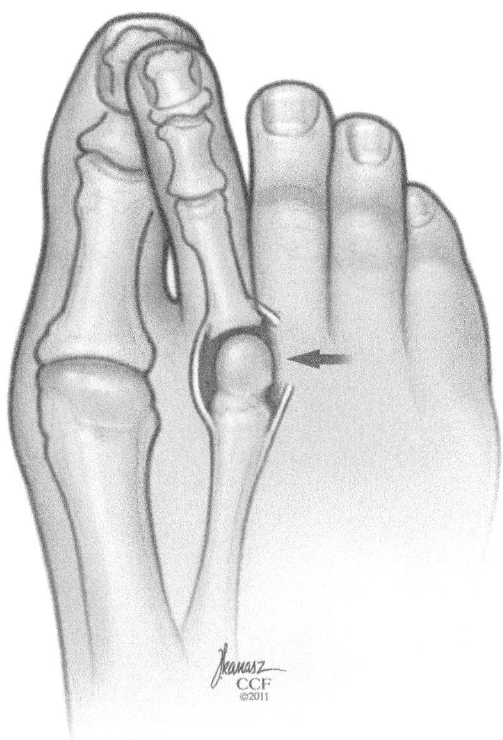

Fig. 2. Failure of lateral collateral ligament leads to progressive varus deformity and ultimately crossover toe. (*Reprinted with permission,* Cleveland Clinic Center for Medical Art & Photography © 2011. All Rights Reserved.)

toes.[1] The most common complaint is pain at the second MTP joint, even in patients with hallux pathology. On physical examination, inspecting the foot readily identifies a dorsomedial subluxation or dislocation of the second toe crossing over the great toe. The affected MTP joint often demonstrates swelling owing to synovitis. The drawer sign is pathognomonic and predictive of instability at the second MTP.[4] The drawer sign is described in which the toe is vertically subluxated to determine relative instability of the joint, akin to a Lachman test of

Table 1
Stages of crossover toe deformity

Grade	Signs
0	Joint pain with swelling of the MTP. Pain with no instability or deformity.
I	Mild instability, positive drawer sign. No deformity.
II	Moderate instability, positive drawer sign. Medial, lateral, dorsal or dorsomedial deformity at the MTP joint.
III	Dislocated MTP, positive drawer sign.
IV	Dislocated MTP with fixed dorsomedial deformity.

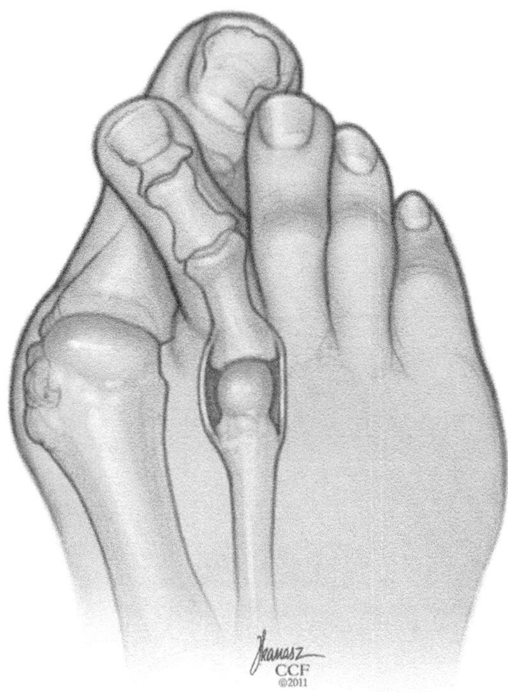

Fig. 3. Crossover toe deformity in conjunction with hallux valgus. (*Reprinted with permission,* Cleveland Clinic Center for Medical Art & Photography © 2011. All Rights Reserved.)

the knee. This stress examination also places strain on the plantar capsule and can elicit pain. The involved toe should be dorsiflexed 25° at the MTP joint during the test and is compared with the contralateral foot as a control. Calluses or intractable plantar keratoses under the second MTP must be identified in these patients as well. A painful dorsal corn over the proximal interphalangeal (PIP) joint as a result of impingement on the toe box may also occur and be a source of discomfort.

Nonoperative Treatment

When approaching the treatment of this deformity, it is prudent to start with nonsurgical measures to alleviate discomfort. Comfortable and well-fitting shoes with a wide toe box large enough to accommodate the deformity is often the first step. Decreasing heel height may also help. Metatarsal pads proximal to the metatarsal head or metatarsal pads built into total contact inserts may be helpful in decreasing pain associated with calluses and intractable plantar keratoses. Taping the toe in a reduced position may help to provide stability to the joint, but does not achieve permanent correction of the deformity. Specific toe cradles or straps may also be effective in cushioning the toe and providing stability, but again are unlikely to achieve any correction of the deformity, only symptomatic relief. A rocker sole or firm insert, such as a metal shank, can be tried to limit motion at the MTP and diminish the pain experienced with walking. Oral anti-inflammatory medications in combination with

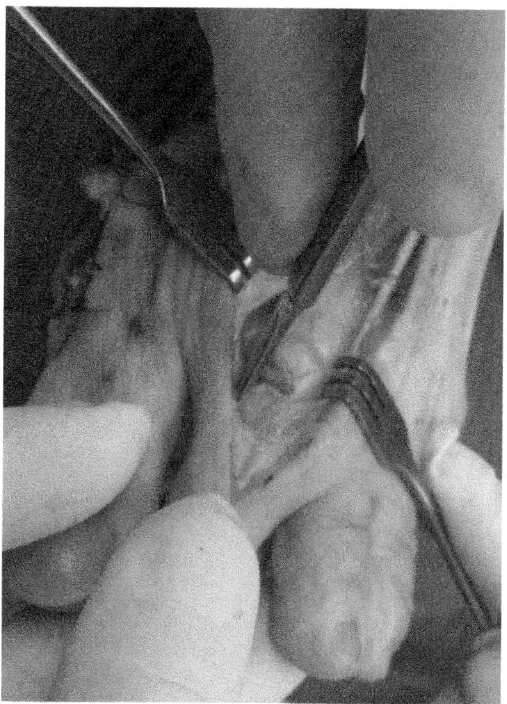

Fig. 4. Release of contracted medial collateral ligament of the MTP joint.

these treatments may provide relief or lessen the symptoms of patients with crossover toe deformity. Often, however, these nonsurgical modalities are not as successful in crossover toe deformity or frank dislocation, as they are for synovitis or mild subluxation.

Surgical Treatment

When conservative measures fail, several surgical options exist for the treatment of crossover toe deformity. When deciding on the approach to surgery, the causative factors of the deformity must be addressed. If a hallux valgus or hallux rigidus is present, these should be addressed at the time of correction to create the appropriate space for the second toe. Soft tissue releases should be among the first steps in correcting the crossover toe deformity. The extensor digitorum longus tendon can be exposed, separated from the extensor hood, and released in a Z-type fashion to be repaired in a lengthened position. The dorsal capsule should then be released to reduce the hyperextension deformity.[5] The contracted medial capsular tissue should also be released (**Fig. 4**). The first lumbrical on the medial aspect of the second toe may also be a deforming force and should be released. The lateral capsular tissue and lateral collateral ligament can be plicated back to the metatarsal head and tightened via a direct soft tissue repair or reattachment with a suture anchor in the metatarsal head. If the toe still is deviated medially, Deland and colleagues[6] described a partial plantar plate release incrementally until axial plane alignment is improved.

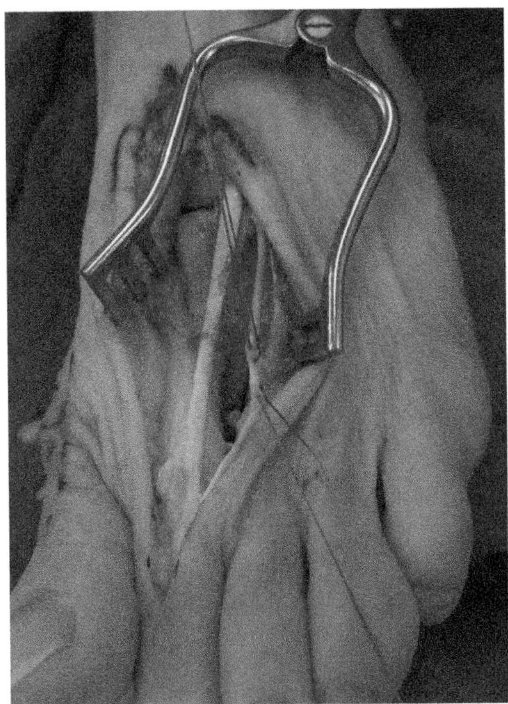

Fig. 5. Nonabsorbable sutures placed proximal and distal to proposed site of EDB tenotomy.

To help stabilize the joint and keep the toe from deviating medially, Haddad and Myerson described a technique to transfer the EDB and redirect its pull lateral and plantar to the second MTP joint. Specifically, they released the MTP joint and carefully dissected out the EDB tendon proximally over the metatarsal, 4 centimeters proximal to MTP joint. Sutures are placed proximally and distally to the tenotomy site (**Fig. 5**) and the EDB is then severed between (**Fig. 6**). The distal stump passes beneath the transverse metatarsal ligament from distal to proximal and lateral to the joint, made easier with use of a curved aneurysm needle (**Fig. 7**). Once the joint is stabilized by a transarticular K-wire, the end of the distal stump is repaired to the proximal stump in an end-to-end fashion[2] (**Fig. 8**). Flexor to extensor tendon transfer (Girdlestone–Taylor procedure) has been described to correct instability in the saggital plane if severe.[2] Barca and Accario[7] have reported good results with flexor digitorum transfer and medial soft tissue release.

If a deformity still persists in spite of these soft tissue procedures, a distal oblique osteotomy of the metatarsal head (such as a Weil or Maceira osteotomy) can be performed to shorten the second metatarsal and relax the soft tissues further (**Fig. 9**). Salvage procedures at the MTP joint include a Duvries resection arthroplasty (reshaping the head with a ronguer at the second MTP) to reduce the toe if dislocated or if the joint is arthritic; other options such as proximal phalangectomy or syndactylization,[8–10] may not relieve pain sufficiently and are not considered aesthetically pleasing to the patient. Amputation of the toe can be a good option in low-demand or elderly individuals who want a "quick fix" without a long recovery. Specific problems of the toe itself are corrected with PIP

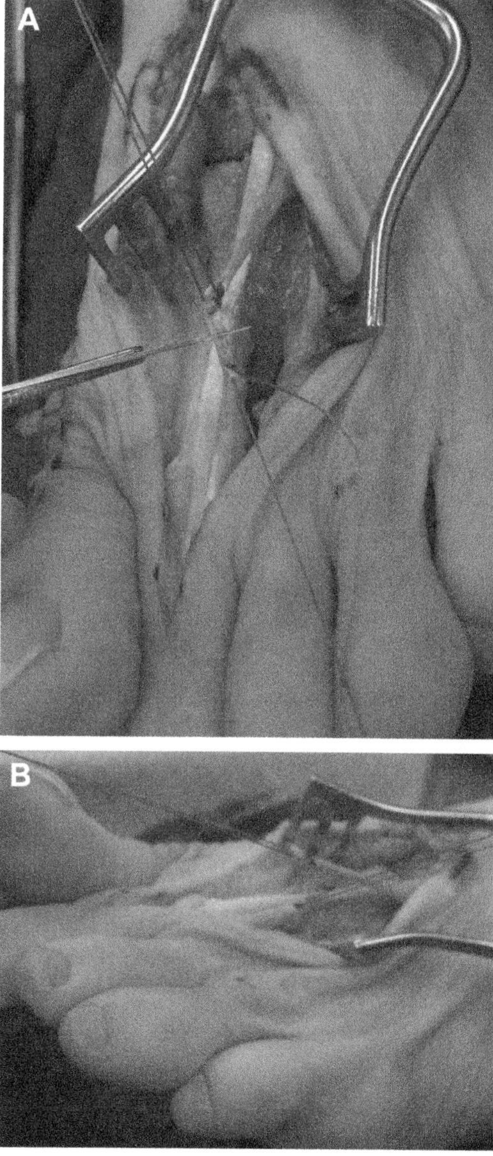

Fig. 6. EDB tendon tenotomy. (*A*) Before release. (*B*) After transaction.

resection arthroplasty, fusion, or Girdlestone–Taylor tendon transfers as covered in other articles in this issue.

Although much of the literature is devoted to the treatment and correction of a medially deviated crossover toe, there can also exist a valgus deviation at the second MTP joint. Typically, this is due to the great toe being in a valgus position. The great toe begins to occupy the space where the second toe resides and the second toe deviates laterally. Similar to the described treatment for a medially deviating crossover toe, the same nonsurgical measures exist. In the event that these fail, typically

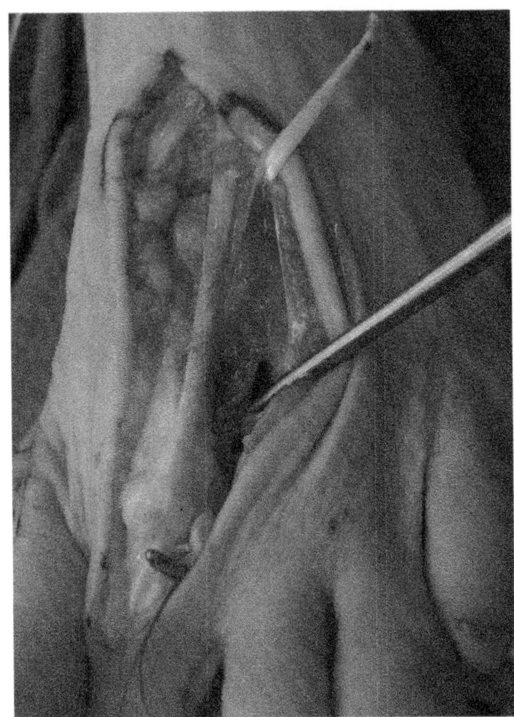

Fig. 7. Passage of EDB distal limb deep to transverse metatarsal with curved aneurysm needle.

soft tissue releases similar to the ones described for crossover toe can be utilized. However, in the case of a valgus toe deformity, the soft tissue structures on the lateral aspect of the joint are contracted and need to be released and the soft tissue structures on the medial aspect of the joint are loosened and can be plicated with a direct soft tissue repair or with suture anchors.

RESULTS

Many procedures have been described, alone or in combination, to treat the crossover toe deformity and for the most part, results of initial treatments are encouraging and successful. Haddad and co-workers[2] noted successful realignment in 14 of 19 of toes with an EDB transfer at an average follow-up of 52 months (**Fig. 10**). Deland and associates[6] looked at 12 patients who had a partial plantar plate release performed in addition to EDB release, EDL lengthening, and capsular releases and all maintained correction of their deformity at 6 to 36 months. Barca and Acciaro[7] have reported good results with flexor digitorum transfer and medial soft tissue release, with 83% of 27 patients (30 toes) having good to excellent results at follow-up. Dhukaram and co-workers[5] performed extensive soft tissue releases and PIP arthroplasty for subluxated MTP deformities. The authors looked at 157 toes in 69 patients; 14% had moderate to severe pain at follow-up. However, correction was good with only two cases of persistent MTP joint instability.[5] Coughlin[1] reported results of surgical correction in 15 toes (11

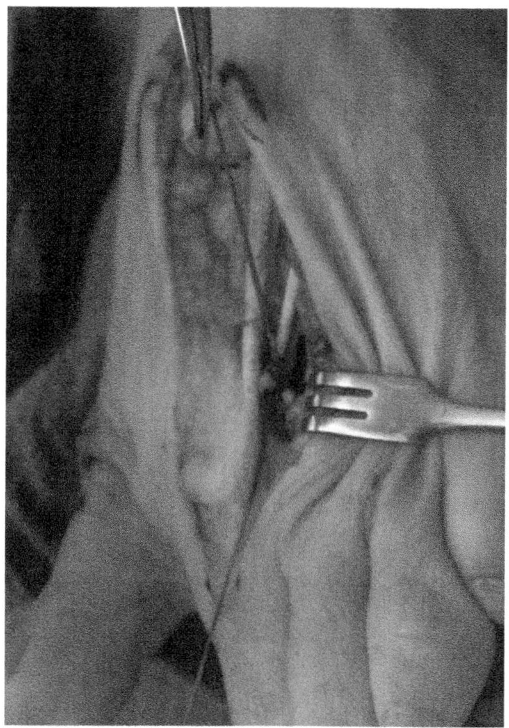

Fig. 8. End-to-end suture repair of EDB tendon.

patients) with a variety of soft tissue releases including extensor tenotomies, flexor tendon transfers, K-wire pinning of the joint, and occasional metatarsal articular resections. They reported 93% good to excellent results with this combination approach. Although these results indicate that good correction and pain relief are likely with index procedures, salvage procedures including proximal phalangectomy, syndactilization, second MTP fusion, and amputation do not yield acceptable results. Conklin and Smith[8] had a 29% dissatisfaction rate after proximal phalangectomy and 40% of patients had some amount of continued pain. Cahill and Connor[9] reported 50% poor results with proximal phalangectomy. Daly and Johnson[10] looked at second and third MTP joints that were treated with proximal phalangectomies and syndactilization. In all, 28% had continued problems with cosmesis, 18% had a recurrent cockup deformity, and 27% noted residual pain.[10] Karlock[11] reported on second MTP arthrodesis to stabilize the dislocated second MTP and reported 10 of 11 good or excellent results.

Complications

Despite good clinical results, complications of operative treatment are present with each surgical option, with many sharing common complications. The more common complications include recurrence of deformity and stiffness of the second MTP joint and second toe. Many patients experience some mild cocking up of the toe (**Fig. 11**). Also, many patients experience continued pain at the second MTP joint, although

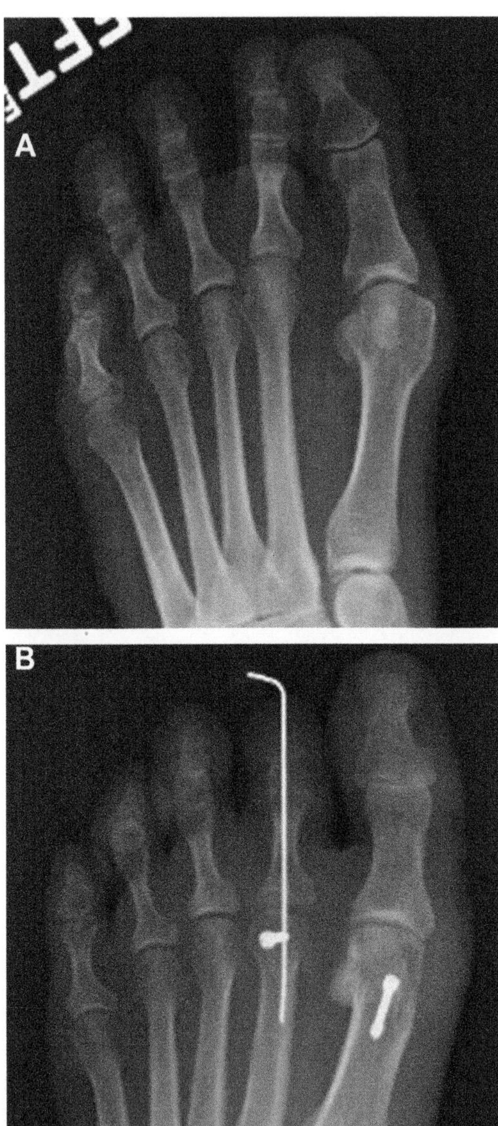

Fig. 9. (*A*) Preoperative radiographs of patient with hallux valgus and crossover toe. (*B*) Postoperative radiographs after bunion correction, EDB transfer and shortening second metatarsal osteotomy.

etiology of this continued pain is often difficult to fully understand. Relative stiffness or joint contracture may cause pain, as can altered mechanics after joint realignment or tendon transfer. Other less common complications include soft tissue atrophy or overcorrection of the toe.

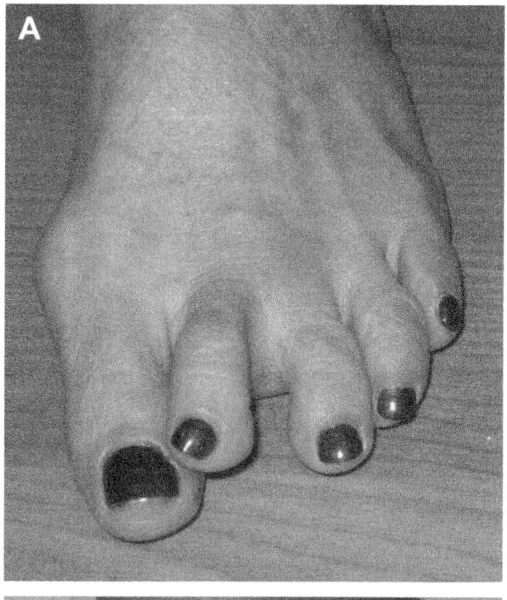

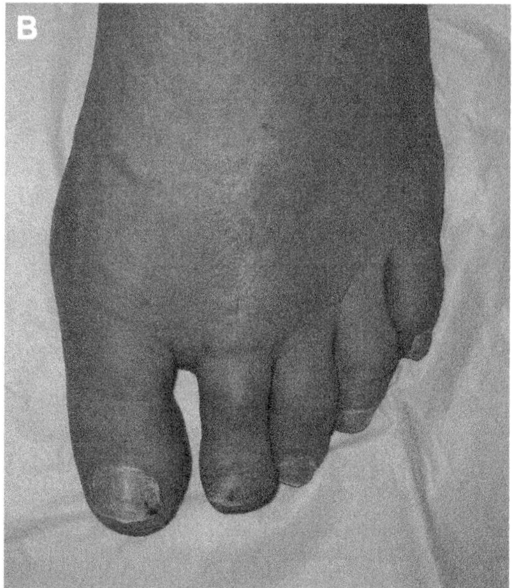

Fig. 10. (*A*) Preoperative clinical image of patient with crossover toe. (*B*) Postoperative image after EDB transfer.

SUMMARY

Second toe problems are among the most common of all forefoot complaints. Its proximity to the hallux combined with limited motion at the second tarsometatarsal joint likely contributes to the second MTP joint being the most common to experience both pain and deformity. Many causes have been linked to this problem, which has lead to many surgical techniques to correct this deformity. Although many techniques

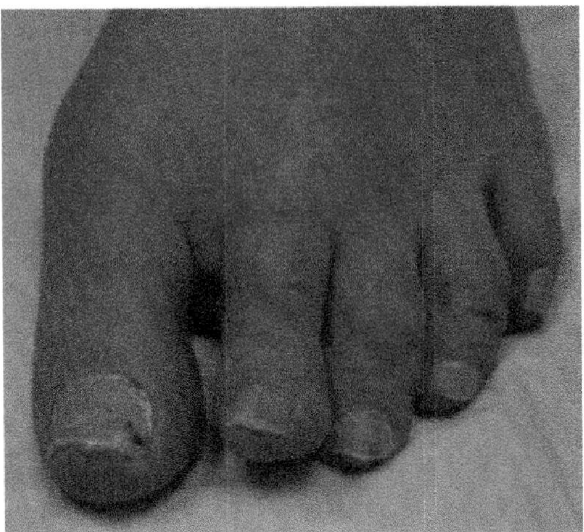

Fig. 11. Residual cock-up deformity of second toe after EDB transfer.

have been described, a systematic approach relying first on soft tissue releases and plication followed by osteotomies as necessary has lead to satisfactory outcomes in the treatment of this difficult problem.

REFERENCES

1. Coughlin MJ. Crossover second toe deformity. Foot Ankle 1987;8:29–39.
2. Haddad SL, Sabbagh RC, Resch S, et al. Results of flexor-to-extensor and extensor brevis tendon transfer for correction of the crossover second toe deformity. Foot Ankle Int 1999;20:781–8.
3. Hatch D, Burns M. An anomalous tendon associated with crossover second toe deformity. J Am Podiatr Med Assoc 1994;84:131–2.
4. Thompson FM, Hamilton WG. Problems of the second metatarsophalangeal joint. Orthopedics 1987;10:83–9.
5. Dhukaram V, Hossain S, Sampath J, et al. Correction of hammer toe with an extended release of the metatarsophalangeal joint. J Bone Joint Surg Br 2002;84:986–90.
6. Deland J, Sung I-H. The medial crossover toe: a cadaveric dissection. Foot Ankle Int 3000;21:375–8.
7. Barca F, Acciaro AL. Surgical correction of crossover deformity of the second toe: a technique for tenodesis. Foot Ankle Int 2004;25:620–4.
8. Conklin MJ, Smith RW. Treatment of the atypical lesser toe deformity with basal hemiphalangectomy. Foot Ankle Int 1994;15:585–94.
9. Cahill BR, Connor DE. A long-term follow-up on proximal phalangectomy for hammer toes. Clin Orthop Relat Res1972;86:191–2.
10. Daly PJ, Johnson KA. Treatment of painful subluxation or dislocation at the second and third metatarsophalangeal joints by partial proximal phalanx excision and subtotal webbing. Clin Orthop Relat Res 1992;278:164–70.
11. Karlock LG. Second metatarsophalangeal joint fusion: a new technique for crossover hammertoe deformity. A preliminary report. J Foot Ankle Surg 2003;42:178–82.

Revision Surgery of the Lesser Toes

Matthew C. Solan, FRCS Tr&Orth*, Mark S. Davies, FRCS Tr&Orth

KEYWORDS

• Revision • Lesser toes • Revision surgery • Toe deformity

A patient once said that her father told her that, "To forget all your troubles you only need to wear a pair of tight shoes." Tight shoes, as even children know, have also been blamed for extreme personality disorders and failure to embrace the Christmas spirit:

The Grinch hated Christmas! The whole Christmas season!

Now, please don't ask why. No one quite knows the reason.

It could be his head wasn't screwed on just right.

It could be, perhaps, that his ***shoes were too tight***.

From "How the Grinch stole Christmas!"

Foot pathology can be extremely debilitating and that the lesser toes are no exception. There are a plethora of operative procedures that can transform the lives of patients suffering from lesser toe disorders. Many lesser toe problems are poorly assessed and many inappropriate surgical procedures are performed. This causes further misery for the patients concerned (**Fig. 1**).

It is acknowledged that extensive literature on revision lesser toe operative techniques and clinical outcomes is somewhat lacking. This chapter describes the authors' approach to the evaluation and treatment of failed lesser toe surgeries. It offers an experienced view of the problems resulting from lesser toe surgery, practical hints on patient evaluation, and an emphasis on revision operative procedures. If carefully planned and executed, surgery can result in a massive improvement in pain and deformity, bringing a much-improved quality of life.

CAUSES OF RECURRENT LESSER TOE PROBLEMS AFTER SURGERY

It is difficult to state what proportion of those patients who undergo lesser toe surgery consider that the treatment has failed. The definition of failure is not straightforward,

London Foot and Ankle Centre, Hospital of St John and St Elizabeth, 80 Grove End Road, London NW8 9NH, UK
* Corresponding author.
E-mail address: Enquiries@footandanklecentre.co.uk

Foot Ankle Clin N Am 16 (2011) 621–645
doi:10.1016/j.fcl.2011.09.002
foot.theclinics.com
1083-7515/11/$ – see front matter

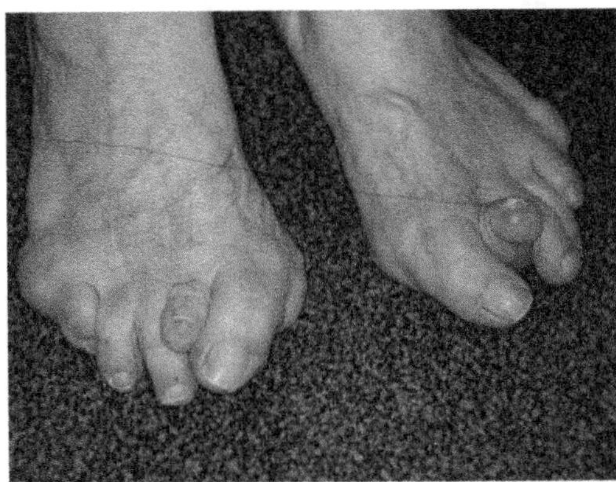

Fig. 1. Toe cripple after poorly performed surgery.

but patient dissatisfaction with the procedure and requirement for revision surgery are 2 good criteria. If the surgeon has not properly explained the nature of the surgery and provided the patient with realistic expectations, then it is easy for the patient to be dissatisfied even if the operative procedure has been executed well. For some patients, a shorter fatter toe or a stiff toe after surgery is simply unacceptable. A thorough preoperative explanation minimizes the chances of postoperative dissatisfaction. In addition, there are some patients who will never be happy, whatever is done. Being able to spot this type of patient (and avoid operative intervention) is a skill worth developing through reflective practice.

Common causes of failure include poorly performed surgery, incorrect choice of procedure, complications (such as infection), failure to predict the sequelae of the surgery, and failure to appreciate a progressive underlying condition. In addition, scars can be unforgiving and nerve and vessel damage can have major repercussions.

A lot of revision toe surgery involves putting right what should have been put right in the first place. Therefore, a review of revision toe surgery needs to include details about the primary surgeries for lesser toes plus all the revision procedures needed to salvage the problems that surgery can create.

PATIENT SELECTION AND TOE CRIPPLES

Before we discuss the pathologies and remedies, it is worth pointing out that patient selection is the key to success when dealing with lesser toe problems, just as it is with all other aspects of surgery. Clearly, proper expectations by the patient are imperative and it is incumbent on the surgeon to inform him or her of what can and cannot be reasonably expected after revision (**Fig. 2**).

Unfortunately, some patients still undergo ill-considered surgery and this causes worsened toe function, pain, and deformity. It is even more unfortunate when these patients are subjected to further mutilating surgery, resulting in a downward spiral (**Fig. 3**). The foot cripple is a well-recognized entity and the "toe cripple" forms a subset of these patients. Most of these individuals become foot obsessed and disabled through no fault of their own. Only rarely do these patients have Munchausen syndrome. The remainder are people who have often been subjected to woeful surgery and their problems have been compounded by more inappropriate surgery. When dealing with such individuals, it is important to realize the misery to which they have been subjected and only offer further surgery if there is

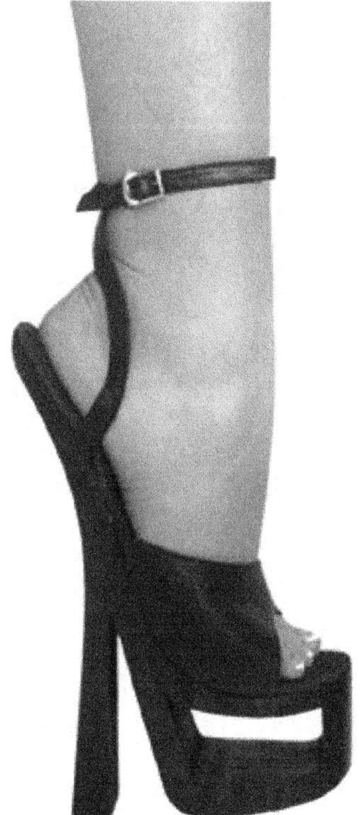

Fig. 2. Patients often harbor unreasonable expectations.

a realistic chance of improving their pain and disability. Successive revision surgeries become more complicated, less predictable, and run the risk of worsening the situation. Often, the most difficult consultations are those wherein the surgeon has to inform the patient that there is nothing more that can be offered to relieve his or her symptoms.

Assessment

As with all foot conditions, a detailed history of the problem and thorough examination are mandatory. Detailed reports of the prior surgery are critical in planning for potential revision. Examination assesses malalignment of the hallux and lesser toes, the presence of prior scars, and localizes points of tenderness (**Fig. 4**). It is unforgiveable to overlook progressive neurologic conditions or fail to diagnose a dysvascular foot before surgery (**Fig. 5**). Equally, inflammatory joint conditions should not be missed and medical records relating to past procedures should be obtained. Ideally, up-to-date, weight-bearing radiographs of the feet should be requested before operative intervention. If any doubt about the vascular status of the limb exists, appropriate vascular evaluation should be performed. Suspicions about neurologic disorders should likewise be acted upon. A thorough clinical examination and nerve conduction studies can be very informative; if there remains any doubt about the nature of the underlying pathology, a formal neurologic consultation should be obtained before any surgery.

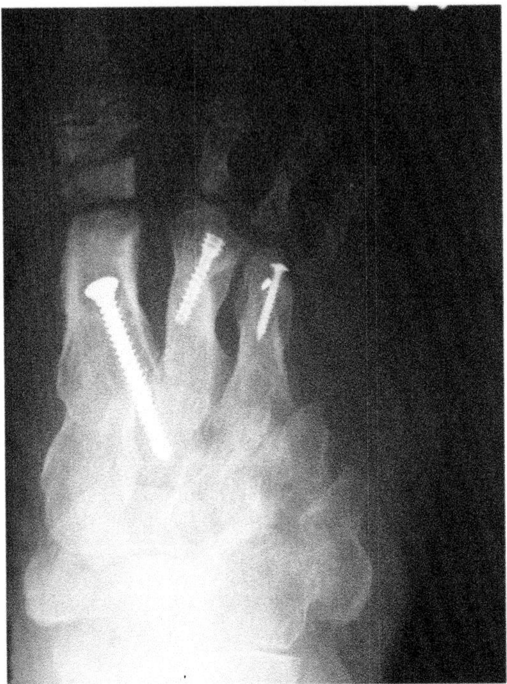

Fig. 3. A painful, deformed, poorly functioning foot after surgical misadventure.

When any patient presents with foot pathology, the treatment options available are to do nothing, modify footwear, utilize various orthotic devices, conduct physical therapy, take medication, and last undergo surgery.[1] This needs to be reiterated whenever a patient presents with recurrent problems with lesser toes. Unfortunately,

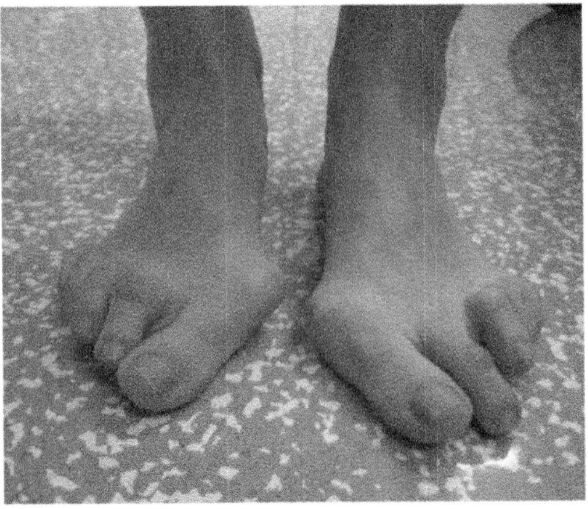

Fig. 4. It is necessary to determine the sources of pain, particularly in the setting of multiple coexisting pathologies.

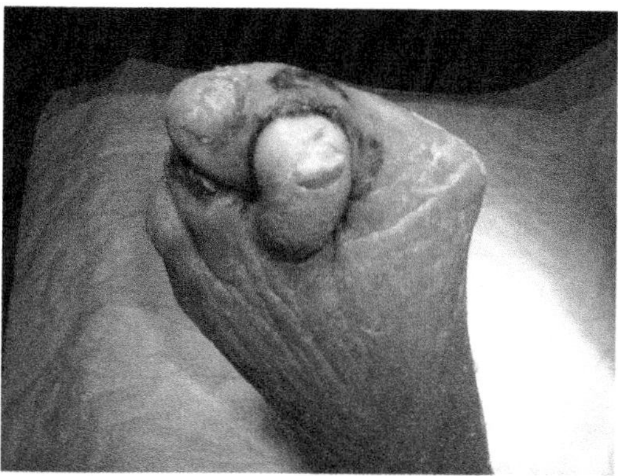

Fig. 5. Vascular insufficiency.

physical therapy and medication only have limited roles in the management of lesser toe deformities and there is a limit to what can be achieved with footwear modification. This is often because patients are unwilling to accept cumbersome orthotics or shoes (**Fig. 6**) and desire a solution that allows the wearing of normal shoes and, particularly in the case of women, fashion shoes. Having said this, if an acceptable orthotic solution can be achieved, then surgery can potentially be avoided. Premetatarsal domes and protective silicone gel toe sleeves can be very effective in relieving pain. Accommodative footwear with an appropriately sized toe box can be found to fit even the most advanced deformity if the patient is willing to comply.

Infection, Ischemia, and Nerve Damage

Before discussing individual pathologies, a review on infection, ischemia, and nerve damage is warranted. Infection can complicate any operative procedure and it is surprising that lesser toe infection is not more common than it is. The lesser toes are prone to infection by virtue of their position in contact with the ground as well as their propensity for swelling. In addition, the lesser toes contain no muscle and are vulnerable to trauma as well as hypoperfusion in cold conditions. Often, venous and

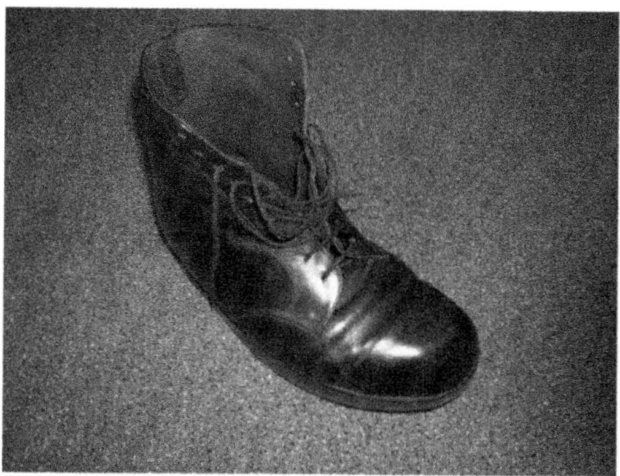

Fig. 6. Wide toe-box, extra-depth footwear.

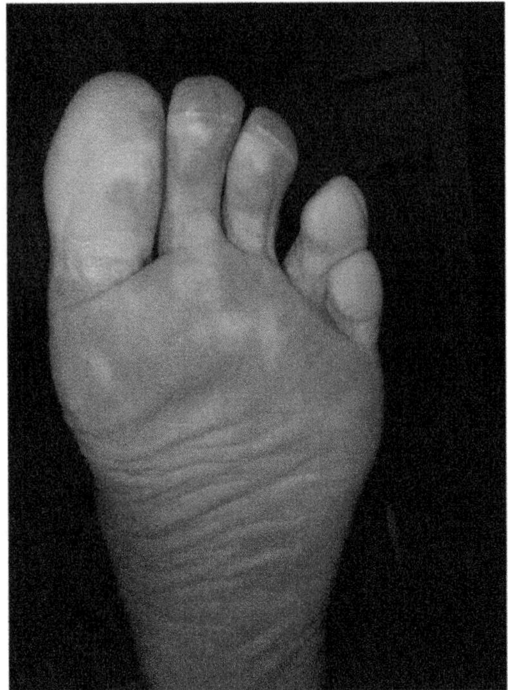

Fig. 7. Raynaud phenomenon.

lymphatic drainage are affected by a surgical incision, as can be the arterial supply to the toe. Additionally, the use of K-wires provides a potential portal for infection.

Particularly in the elderly and in smokers, the risk of toe ischemia needs to be considered before embarking upon surgery. Patients with vasculitic conditions and Raynaud phenomenon need to be carefully assessed preoperatively (**Fig. 7**). The presence or absence of peripheral pulses needs to be documented and, if absent or weak, appropriately investigated before elective surgery is undertaken. The blood supply to the toes needs to be considered when making surgical incisions and soft tissue handling must be gentle to minimize the risk of injury to the vessels. Incisions on the sides of the toes, in the region of the neurovascular bundle, should be avoided. A dorsal incision alone is safe but when combined with other incisions increases the risk of ischemia. Another cause of toe ischemia is damage to the common digital arteries in adjacent web spaces. This may occur during simultaneous second and third space neuroma surgery or with multiple lesser metatarsal osteotomies. Under no circumstances should 2 adjacent neuromata be removed or 2 adjacent metatarsophalangeal joints (MTPJs) released through 2 parallel incisions on the dorsum of the foot (**Fig. 8**). In the case of a dislocated MTPJ, reduction of the toe can lead to stretching of the vessels and nerves as a result of acute lengthening, especially in the elderly.

It is not uncommon at the end of an operative procedure on a lesser toe to see a white, lifeless toe, usually as a result of arterial spasm induced by cold, traction on the vascular structures, and soft tissue trauma (**Fig. 9**). If the toe remains white for more than a few minutes, then the surgeon must ensure that the dressing is not constrictive or compressing the neurovascular bundles of the digit. If the toe remains

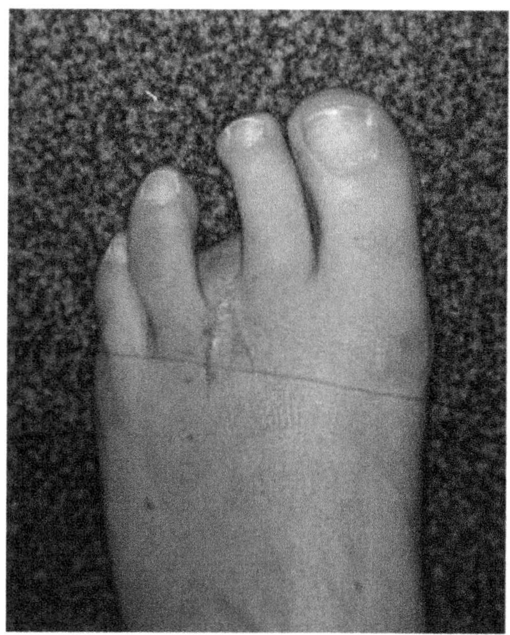

Fig. 8. It is important to avoid parallel incisions placed too close together.

white, the patient should be appropriately warmed and the limb lowered relative to the heart until reperfusion occurs. This can be performed in the recovery room and the foot warmed with use of a heating lamp. Topical use of nitroglycerine paste has been used anecdotally to promote vessel relaxation and reperfusion with frequent success. If the toe has been held with a wire and the toe remains pale for a prolonged period ($>$1 hour) despite these initial measures, then the authors advise removal of the wire and loose taping of the toe to the adjacent digit: It is better to lose the toe's correction than the toe itself. Should this fail to resolve the problem, an urgent vascular consultation should be sought. In the authors' experience, this has never been required. Often, after lesser toe surgery, the toe develops a disconcerting, bluish hue owing to venous congestion. This most often resolves over a period of several minutes, but can take several hours or even days. In such circumstances, the limb should be kept horizontal, rather than elevated or dependent, and the patient should not be excessively warmed, because this encourages vasodilation and therefore further venous congestion.

Nerve damage can lead to long-term pain and misery for a patient and it is incumbent upon the surgeon to minimize the risk of neural damage. This is best achieved by careful placement of incisions, gentle soft tissue handling, and careful needle placement during the administration of local anesthetic blocks. If a traumatic neuroma of a lesser toe occurs, it can be very distressing to the patient. If nonoperative strategies fail to resolve the problem, then repair of the nerve by a surgeon familiar with such surgery may be considered. Burial of the neuroma into bone or muscle are alternative procedures that are likely to be more helpful.

Severe infection or ischemia that do not resolve ultimately result in the need for amputation. Intractable nerve pain can also lead to amputation, but still may not lead to full resolution of pain.

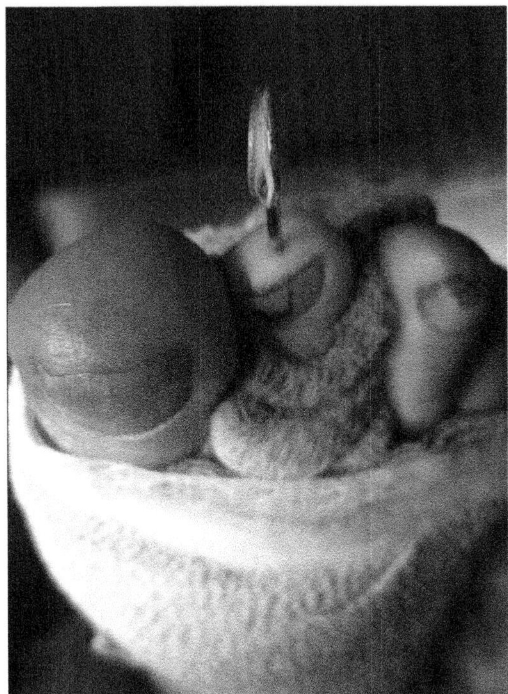

Fig. 9. Dysvascular toe postoperatively.

The Failed Mallet Toe

The commonest cause of a failed mallet toe is an isolated tightness of one of the slips of the flexor digitorum longus (FDL) tendon. Mallet toe may also develop after a proximal interphalangeal (PIP) joint fusion, again owing to tightness of the FDL. The treatment of recurrent mallet toe depends on the degree of flexibility of the distal interphalangeal (DIP) joint. If the deformity is flexible and completely correctible with the ankle and MTPJs held plantar flexed, then an FDL tenotomy is the operation of choice. For a fixed deformity, a tenotomy is unsuccessful if performed in isolation, but may be useful in conjunction with a bony procedure. The authors believe that a DIP joint excision arthroplasty is a superior procedure to a DIP fusion. K-wire stabilization is preferred to screw fixation. A thin wire (1.2 mm) is sufficient and retained for 6 weeks. Occasionally after a bony procedure, an iatrogenic delta phalanx can be created. This is best addressed by performing further bone resection parallel to the joint surface of the terminal phalanx, thereby straightening the toe. Partial amputation of the toe is very much a last resort.

The Failed Hammer Toe

A patient may be dissatisfied with hammer toe surgery for several reasons. Persisting stiffness, pain, and deformity are the commonest complaints (**Fig. 10**). Hammer toes before surgery are often stiff and many of the operative procedures deployed to "correct" the deformity produces a further degree of stiffness. Preoperatively, the surgeon should explain that stiffness is a likely consequence of surgery, especially with a PIP fusion. If the patient is unwilling to tolerate some degree of stiffness, an

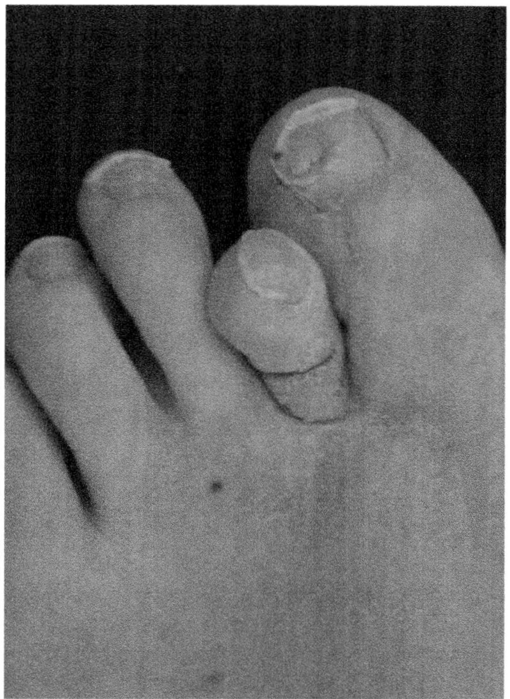

Fig. 10. Flail toe.

alternative procedure such as an excision arthroplasty might be considered. Somewhat surprisingly, despite the nonunion rate of PIP fusion being as high as 50%, nonunion is usually painless and tolerated quite well. Many patients undergoing PIP joint fusion will develop a DIP joint flexion contracture, which may be flexible or fixed. The flexible deformity can be corrected by a flexor tenotomy in the plantar skin crease. If the deformity is fixed, the options are to convert the PIP joint fusion to an excision arthroplasty with or without a flexor tenotomy. In an attempt to maintain length when converting a PIP joint fusion to an excision arthroplasty, soft tissue interposition can be attempted. An alternative is to perform a DIP joint excision arthroplasty with or without a flexor tenotomy. DIP joint fusion often results in nonunion so an excision arthroplasty is preferred (**Fig. 11**). It is important not to overshorten the toe, not only for cosmetic reasons, but also because a flail toe is to be avoided if at all possible. The authors do not use flexor to extensor tendon transfers as a flexor tenotomy is as effective at correcting flexible deformities and is technically easier to perform (**Fig. 12**). In addition, flexor to extensor tendon transfer surgery is frequently associated with marked stiffness and creation of a reverse (ie, swan neck) deformity.[2] Given that flexor to extensor tendon transfer is for the correction of flexible deformities, it is not well-suited for most revision hammer toe operations.

Swelling after hammertoe surgery is common and takes 6 to 12 months to settle. Persistent swelling, particularly in association with excessive erythema or a nonhealing wound, suggests infection. This is a rare occurrence, but probably occurs more frequently in patients with inflammatory joint disease, particularly those taking immunosuppressive, disease-modifying drugs. Appropriate imaging (**Fig. 13**) and

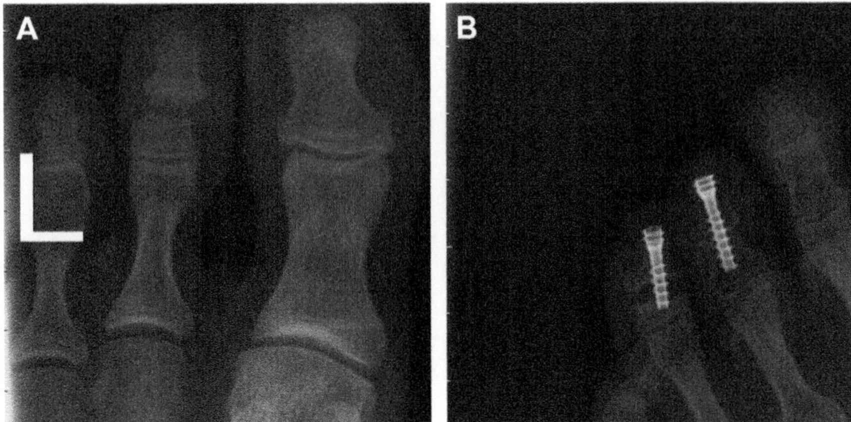

Fig. 11. (*A, B*) Excision arthroplasty is preferred to fixation.

biopsy and culture specimens should be obtained where deep bone infection is suspected. Treatment, as for any osteomyelitis, involves debridement and appropriate antibiotics until the toe is quiescent and all clinical and laboratory indicators of infection are back to normal. If infection cannot be controlled, the toe should be amputated, leaving as much length as possible but ensuring that all infected, necrotic tissue is removed.

If a toe has been excessively shortened, it is difficult to regain length and only rarely should an attempt be made to do so. However, there are circumstances where a flail toe is unacceptable to the patient and an attempt at stabilization with a bone graft and transfixion wire is worth consideration.[3,4] It is usually easier, however, to improve the appearance by shortening other toes to harmonize the appearance of the foot (**Fig. 14**). In such circumstances, shortening should be done within the toe itself rather than shortening the metatarsal. This can be achieved by middle phalangeal diaphyseal shortening or through a DIP joint excision arthroplasty, providing that the middle phalanx is long enough. The middle phalanges of the second and third toes are

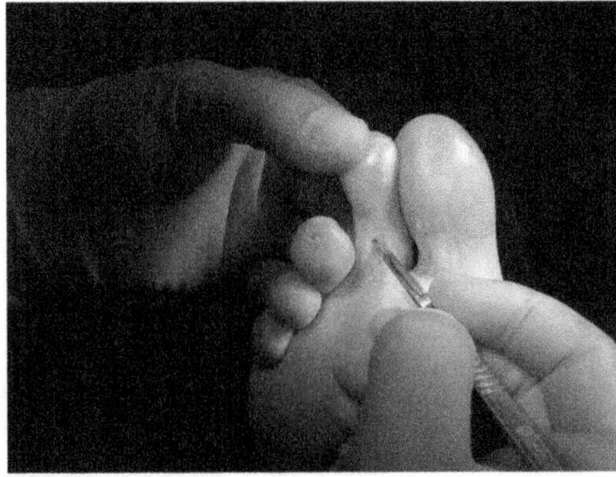

Fig. 12. Flexor tenotomy.

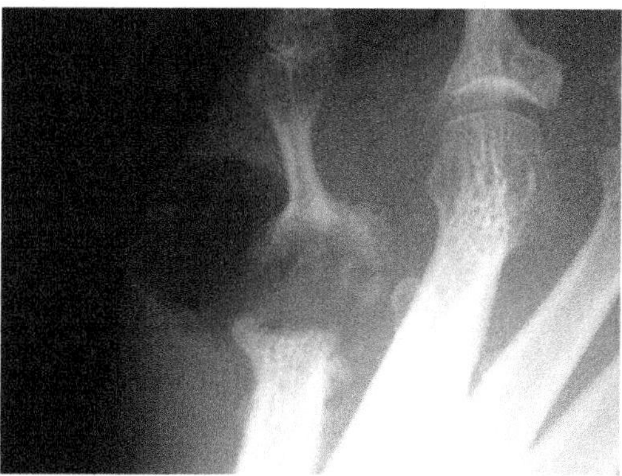

Fig. 13. Deep infection, noteworthy for bony erosion and subcutaneous air.

usually long enough, whereas those of the fourth and fifth are not. If the middle phalanx is too short, then a PIP joint excision can be performed or a diaphyseal shortening, which can be carried out using a minimally invasive technique (**Fig. 15**). The most common source of dissatisfaction after lesser toe surgery is pain; often, this is as a result of persisting deformity, with pressure or friction over a bony prominence. The most common deformities after hammer toe surgery are MTPJ extension and recurrent hyperflexion deformity of the PIP joint.

MTPJ contracture can be extremely rigid. An isolated extensor tenotomy would be ineffective at correcting the deformity. To achieve correction, a full capsular incision and release from the dorsum is required, along with extensor tendon lengthening.[5] In addition, to achieve MTPJ flexion, adhesions and scar tissue should be released from the plantar aspect of the joint using a McGlamary elevator and gentle manipulation. Flexion deformity of the PIP joint can be addressed by revision fusion or a flexor

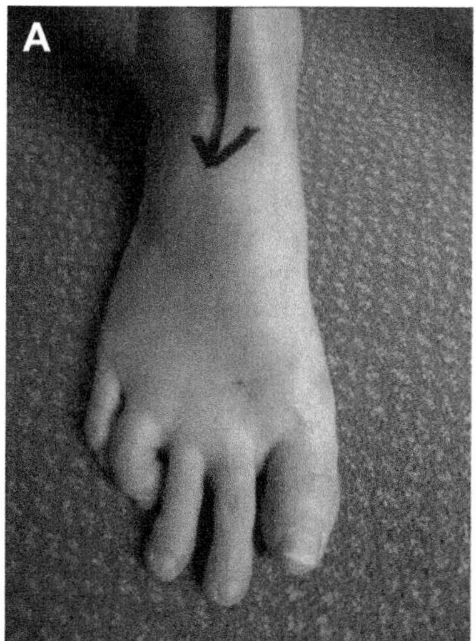

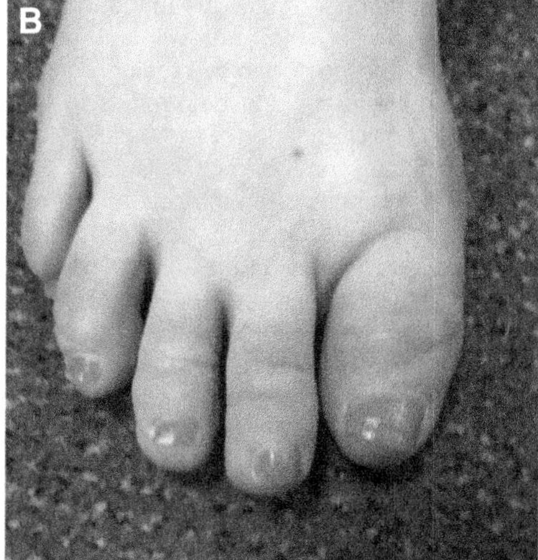

Fig. 14. Restoration of more equalized relative lengths.

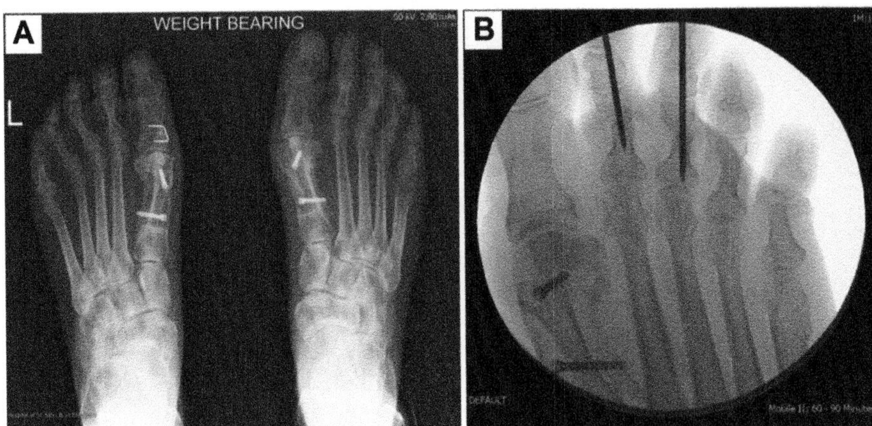

Fig. 15. (*A, B*) Minimally invasive technique with eventual union.

tendon tenotomy. The latter can be carried out through a plantar approach or, if the PIP joint has been opened, through the joint, taking care to avoid the neurovascular bundle. Occasionally, a hammer toe is associated with a highly unstable MTPJ with subluxation or dislocation. When the MTPJ is easily reducible, it can be effectively treated with what is known in the UK as the Cobb 2 procedure, because it was the brainchild of Nigel Cobb, who popularized his unpublished technique. It stabilizes the MTPJ and can be carried out in association with PIP joint surgery at the same time, if required. A dorsal incision is made over the MTPJ and either the extensor digitorum longus or extensor digitorum brevis tendon is divided approximately 5 cm proximal to the MTPJ. A small notch is made on the dorsum of the proximal phalanx to prevent subluxation of the tendon. A drill hole is made from the dorsal aspect of the metatarsal neck into and through the metatarsal head. The tendon is then pulled through the drill hole and sutured to the soft tissue on the dorsum of the metatarsal. A K-wire may be required for temporary stability. It is worth pointing out that if the drill hole is too plantar, it is difficult to pass the tendon through the drill hole. Conversely, if the drill hole is too dorsal, the joint will not be anatomically reduced. **Fig. 16** shows preoperative and postoperative radiographs of a Cobb 2 procedure.

Other problems include deformities in the frontal plane, which can usually be corrected by a combination of soft tissue release and/or appropriate osteotomy of the proximal phalanx and K-wire stabilisation.[6] Putting right what should have been done the first time round is often the solution for a problematic lesser toe that has already been operated upon. One very good example of this is when bone resection has been performed inaccurately. **Fig. 17** shows poor technique of PIP arthroplasty, corrected by simple revision bone removal in a 77-year-old woman. Another useful method of correcting coronal plane deformities is to use a basal closing-wedge osteotomy of the proximal phalanx with K-wire stabilization.

Flail toes are extremely difficult to salvage, but if an arthrodesis can be achieved this is preferable to amputation. Occasionally a partial amputation can be an acceptable solution[1,7] (**Fig. 18**). Syndactylization has been described as a salvage procedure for flail toe, but is cosmetically displeasing and the authors have no experience with its use.[8] It is best to prevent flail toe in the first place by avoiding excessive bone resection, particularly from the proximal phalanx, and to use some form of stabilization for 4 to 6 weeks thereafter, usually with a K-wire.

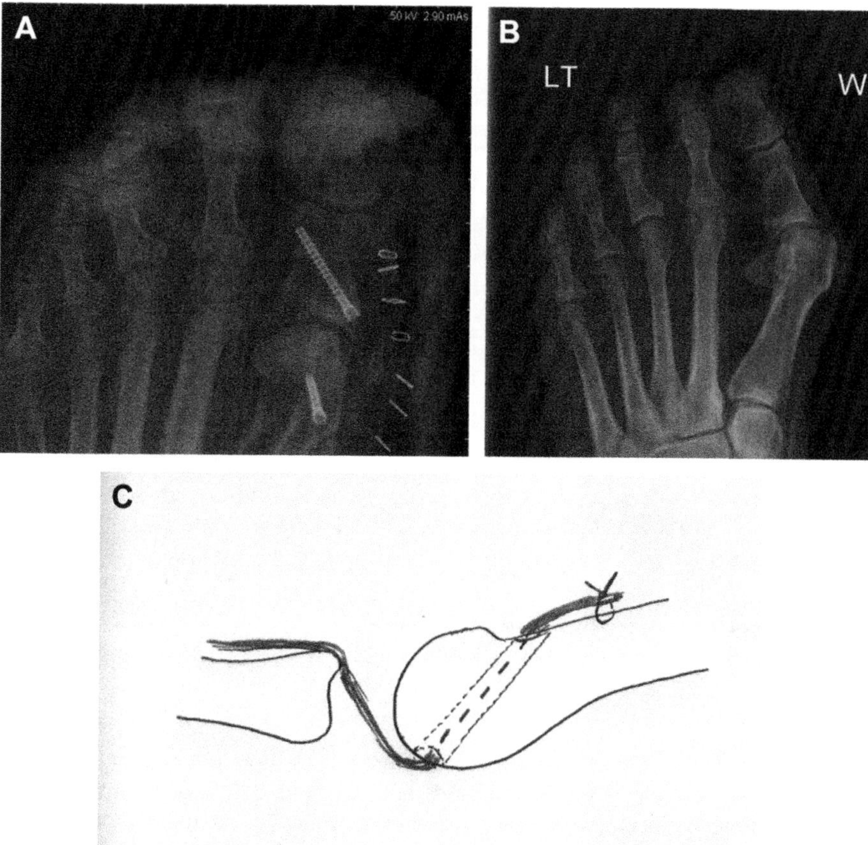

Fig. 16. *(A–C)* Cobb 2 procedure.

One particularly difficult case to salvage is the failed hemiphalangectomy.[9] Lesser toe hemiphalangectomy is still an operation that is performed quite frequently as part of the Stainsby procedure. This is a procedure best reserved for rheumatoid patients and should rarely, if ever, be performed in isolation for a lesser toe deformity. Hemiphalangectomy can result in severe deformity and floppiness of the toe; it can be very difficult, if not impossible, to revise. Occasionally, a soft tissue release can help, but it is by no means guaranteed to improve matters. The Cobb 2 procedure can be helpful to improve the excessively dorsiflexed position that the toe frequently adopts, but controlling deviation in the frontal plane is difficult. A temporary K-wire is almost essential under such circumstances, but does not guarantee maintenance of toe position. Sometimes, amputation needs to be considered, but the patient needs to realize that this is an irreversible operation that can lead to progressive deformities of the adjacent lesser toes.

The Failed Clawtoe

Much of what has been outlined on failed hammer toe surgery also applies to failed clawtoe surgery. It is necessary to correct any residual or recurrent PIP deformity

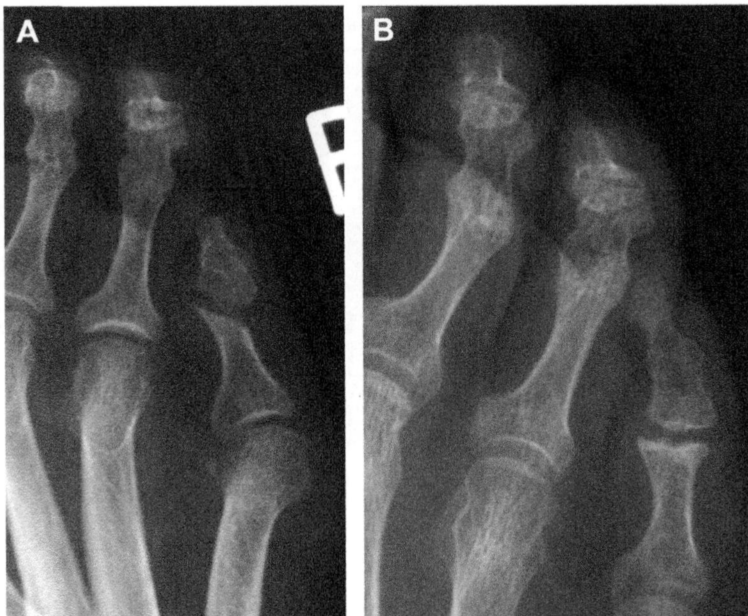

Fig. 17. (*A, B*) Bone spike successfully revised.

along with the MTPJ. Clawtoes differ from hammer toes more in terms of pathogenesis than in actual deformity. Hammer toes are often found in isolation, the majority being second toes; the cause is usually mechanical. Clawtoes are usually multiple and bilateral and have an underlying neurologic cause. As such, clawtoes may recur with time owing to progressive neurologic disease, even if proper surgery was initially performed. Attempts to correct clawtoes with simple flexor tenotomies alone can result in great symptomatic relief, but deformity recurs. Sometimes, it is worth repeating the flexor tenotomy, but often a revision bony procedure such as excision arthroplasty or PIP fusion may be required in addition. Also, for cases of fixed MTPJ hyperextension, aggressive joint releases and extensor lengthening may be required in addition to procedures on the toes. Modified Jones' procedure (the so-called Hibbs procedure) for the lesser toes has been described for the neurologic deformity, using the extensor tendons through or under the metatarsal necks, although the authors believe that few deformities require this surgery. More extensive discussion of revision MTPJ problems follows.

It is worth pointing out that in cases of metatarsalgia and cavus deformity, Weil's osteotomies should be avoided. There is an inevitable, albeit mild, lowering of the metatarsal head and shortening with the Weil's osteotomy. In the cavus foot, this leads to worsening of deformity and increased loads under the metatarsal heads. For such deformities, more proximal bony and soft tissue procedures are required, but these fall outside the scope of this article.

METATARSOPHALANGEAL JOINT PROBLEMS

Deformity at the MTPJ is of paramount importance when dealing with lesser toe symptoms in both the primary and revision operative situation. In the toe, it is the most

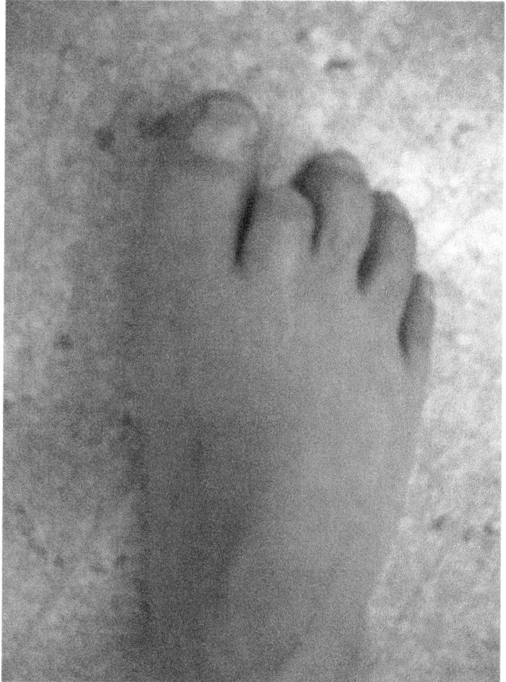

Fig. 18. Partial amputation.

proximal joint and so even mild deformity has a pronounced impact on the shape of the digit and thus symptoms more distally. Improper treatment, with failure to address extension contracture of the MTPJ, is the most commonly encountered reason for failed treatment of claw or hammer toe. Deformity or persistent pain can also occur after prior surgery for other MTP pathologies, including synovitis, crossover toe, or Freiberg's infraction. Stiffness at the joint is also a common complication and every effort should be made to prevent it. Proper rehabilitation and stretching not only helps to ensure the desired outcome after revision surgery, but may be employed after primary operative treatment.

CLASSIFY THE PRESENTING COMPLAINTS

Classifying the nature of the MTPJ problem helps to ensure an individualized treatment plan. The MTPJ may give rise to symptoms either because of pathology at the joint directly producing pain, or through deformity at the joint causing indirect symptoms. A third category of problems relate to other parts of the foot as indirect consequence of an MTPJ problem. Transfer of load to the third MTPJ after otherwise successful treatment of a second toe problem is one such example. Residual second MTPJ pain, altered gait and diffuse lateral forefoot symptoms is another commonly encountered scenario.

MTPJ Problems

Direct MTPJ problems can occur in a well-aligned toe, and include mechanical synovitis, osteochondritis, degenerative, and inflammation. MTPJ deformities include

Box 1
Assessment of MTPJ problems

MTPJ pain with no deformity

Intrinsic: Mechanical, degenerative, or inflammatory synovitis

Extrinsic: Lesser MT shaft stress response, interdigital neuritis or bursitis

MTPJ pain and deformity

Sagittal plan (extension): With or without dorsal subluxation

Coronal plane (varus/valgus)

Mixed (rotation)

Exacerbating factors

Forefoot: Hallux valgus or rigidus; neighboring lesser MTPJ pain

Midfoot: Hypermobility of TMT; degenerative TMT pathology

Hindfoot: Joint stiffness of pain leading to altered gait

Proximal: Gastrocnemius or Achilles contracture, knee malalignment

Other: Body mass index, vascular supply, neuropathy

plantar plate rupture, fat pad migration, and MT head pressure. Indirect MTJP problem manifest AS Symptoms distal to MTPJ secondary to deformity at MTPJ. A sagittal deformity produces dorsal PIP joint callosity or toe tip pain/extensor lag. A coronal plane deformity produces pressure symptoms or overlapping toes. Other parts of foot can also be affected, and include load transfer to neighboring MTPJ because of MTPJ pain and abnormal gait. Direct problems may be divided into pain from degenerative or inflammatory joint disease with normal joint alignment, and pain from the MTPJ with abnormal joint alignment. Deformity may be in the sagittal plane or the coronal plane. Where these 2 coexist, axial rotation is almost certainly present too.

Indirect problems occur with abnormal MTPJ alignment, causing pain not at the MTPJ itself but more distally in the toe. Corns and callosities form as a result of pressure against the neighboring digit (with MTPJ varus or valgus), the floor (toe tip pain with fixed MTPJ flexion or extensor lag) or the toe box of an enclosed shoe (at the PIP joint with extension deformity at the MTPJ). **Box 1** summarizes these various categories.

Direct Pain in the Absence of MTP Deformity

Transfer of load to the lesser rays (particularly the second and third) in patients with first ray problems gives rise to lesser ray problems of one sort or another. Whether a particular foot develops lesser MTPJ synovitis, degenerative arthrosis at the MTPJ, a stress fracture of the metatarsal shaft, or a degenerative change at the tarsometatarsal joint is not predictable. The length of time that it takes for lesser ray problems to appear after the onset of hallux pathology is not well understood either. What experience does tell us, however, is that lesser toe problems eventually arise and that these secondary problems manifest more quickly in the presence of “unfavorable features,” including relatively long lesser metatarsals, shortening of the gastrocnemius, and a high body mass index. Identifying and addressing these features before surgery or revision surgery is important.

Direct Pain with Deformity at the MTPJ

Residual deformity at the joint, whether in the sagittal plane or varus/valgus, results in pain underneath the lesser MT head. Correcting this is imperative if the revision surgery is to be successful. In practice, this direct MTPJ pain is nearly always eclipsed by the indirect (and more visible) symptoms in the more distal part of the toe (eg, dorsal callosity at the PIP joint). Addressing these "obvious" problems only is not advisable because of the high risk of persistent symptoms from the MPTJ.

MANAGEMENT

Thorough assessment of the presenting symptoms is essential for successful treatment. Straightening the toe with a PIP joint excision arthroplasty or fusion will not help the patient whose main complaint is of pain from degenerative changes at the MTPJ. Similarly, even a full and thorough lesser toe procedure will have a disappointing outcome for the patient in whom the first ray is the root cause of poor foot biomechanics. Only after a full assessment and consideration of all nonoperative treatments should plans for revision surgery be made. Weight loss, activity modification, analgesia, orthotics (either corrective or accommodative), shoe modification, and toe props/pads are all relatively simple and risk free management strategies. Very few patients have genuinely exhausted all nonoperative avenues. On the other hand, cumbersome footwear and orthotics are a "hard sell" if surgery offers a potential long-term solution.

When deciding upon the best strategy for revision surgery, it is important to consider what has already been attempted at the MPTJ. Frequently, the MTPJ will not have been addressed during the index operative procedure at all. For the revision surgeon, this is the ideal scenario. Where surgery has been undertaken, a full analysis of the reasons for failure ensures that the appropriate procedure is selected and give best chance of successful revision. Was the first procedure appropriate? If so, was it performed properly and was the rehabilitation sufficient? If the first treatment was not appropriate is the main problem now in the bone or the soft tissues? Have coexisting foot problems conspired to ruin the result of the first operation? Are there factors beyond the foot itself that should be included in the treatment? Is the MTPJ reduced or dorsally subluxed?

To successfully deal with the MTPJ, a full range of bony and soft tissue procedures are required. No single recipe answers all problems. In an area of orthopaedic surgery, where there is very little science, heavy reliance is placed upon the "art" of selecting the right procedure in the right patient at the right time.

Soft Tissue Procedures

The most common soft tissue complication after MTPJ surgery is residual extension contracture at the joint, often with dorsal subluxation. This may be due to undercorrection or recurrence of the deformity. The latter most frequently arises as a consequence of inadequate rehabilitation. Scarring of the dorsal soft tissues produces dorsal translation and extension. Because the plantar plate is not normal, the main static restraint against extension is easily overcome. The result is a "floating" toe, which has inadequate ground contact and an excess of pressure at the metatarsal head.

MPTJ Release

All too often, the MTPJ is either ignored or an isolated extensor digitorum longus tenotomy is performed as part of the primary surgery. A soft tissue release for significant MTPJ extension should include lengthening of both of the extensor tendons, circumferential release of the joint capsule (down to but not including the flexor tendons),[5] and release of the plantar scar tissue under the MT head. In revision surgery, scarring around the joint is considerable and careful dissection is required to ensure that all contracted tissues are properly released. Only if there is residual tendency for the MTP to sublux (tested in a simulated weight bearing position) should consideration be given to additional procedures. It is, however, essential to anticipate and plan ahead. If the extensor apparatus is to be used for a tendon transfer or tenodesis procedure, then careful preservation at the time of soft tissue release is important. A Cobb 2 interposition arthroplasty is much more difficult to perform if the extensor longus has already been lengthened or if a Weil osteotomy has been performed as part of this revision operation.

Tendon Transfer

Flexor to extensor tendon transfer is not commonly used by the authors because this supposed joint-preserving surgical option leads to PIP joint stiffness as well as stiffness of the MTPJ generally.[2] Extensor tendon transfers can be used to help rebalance deformity—especially coronal plane deviation. Split extensor transfer of the long extensor (from the opposite side to the direction of deformity) is secured as distally as possible to maximize the corrective force. For example, one third of the extensor digitorum longus can be detached distally and rerouted to the extensor digitorum communis of the second toe distal to the MTPJ. In a varus deformity, the extensor digitorum brevis can be transferred beneath the lateral intermetatarsal ligament, mimicking the better known procedure described for the correction of hallux varus.[10]

Interposition Arthroplasty

Although excision arthroplasty of the lesser MTPJs is a reliable procedure for end-stage rheumatoid arthritis, resection of the MT head or base of the proximal phalanx is best avoided if possible. Where there is pain from degenerative arthritis of a lesser MTPJ, interposition arthroplasty provides pain relief. Resection of a small amount of the base of the proximal phalanx and the osteophytes from the MT head is performed at the same time as suturing the extensor hood to the flexor tendons, or performing a formal Cobb 2 procedure.

Tenodesis Procedures

The Cobb 2 procedure, as described, is both an interposition arthroplasty and a tenodesis. Its strength lies in the reduction of dorsal displacement of the toe. Attention to technical detail is important, and in a revision situation the availability of sufficient quantity of extensor tendon is a potential limitation. Proximal division of the long extensor should be as proximal as possible to allow reattachment after passage through the metatarsal head drill hole (≥2.5 mm in diameter).

Plantar Plate Repair

Reattachment of the plantar plate has been reported in the literature, but there are more cadaver studies than clinical ones.[11–13] Restoring the integrity of the principal restraint to dorsal subluxation is clearly a logical and appealing concept. A reliable and technically reproducible means of reattaching the abnormal plantar plate is not, however, yet a reality.

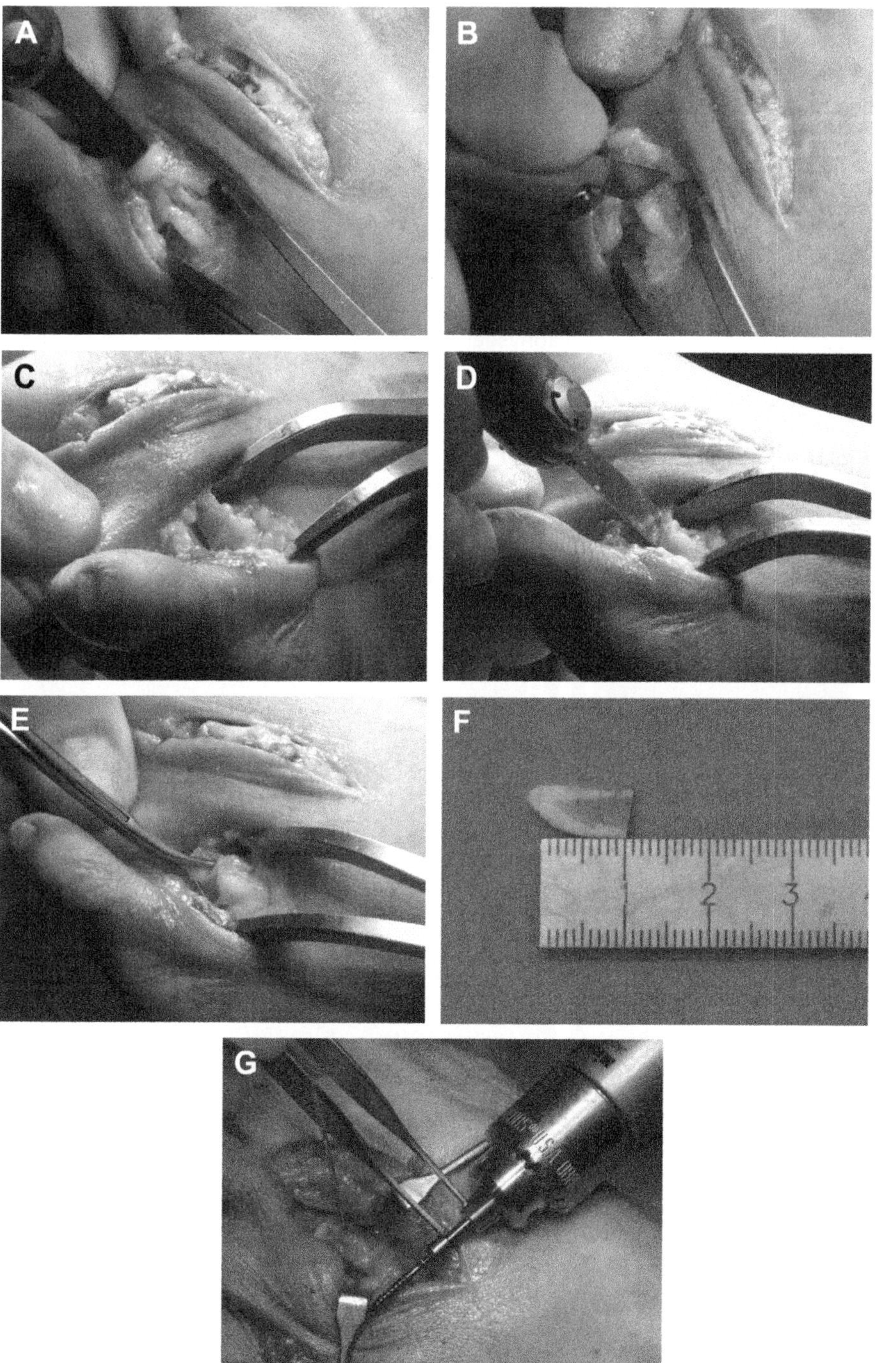

Fig. 19. (*A–G*) Double cut for Weil metatarsal osteotomy.

BONY PROCEDURES

Osteotomy

For more than 10 years, the Weil lesser metatarsal neck osteotomy, has been a widely used means of shortening lesser metatarsals.[14,15] The philosophy is that established soft tissue contractures can be relaxed through shortening of the bone. Leaving the toe itself long retains both function and cosmoses. This shortening is likely to mean that (multiple) Weil osteotomies are required to balance the weight bearing function of the forefoot. In some cases all 4 lesser metatarsals are shortened, even if they are symptom free. Advantages of the Weil procedure are that it allows precise shortening and that the osteotomy is fixed internally. It is a metaphysical osteotomy and so heals reliably. These features are important when the alternatives of a Helal (uncontrolled oblique sliding) osteotomy or diaphyseal shortening osteotomy are considered. There are, however, drawbacks with the Weil osteotomy. Poor technique can result in inadvertent lowering of the metatarsal head.[16] This results in residual discomfort under the MTPJ. Shortening of a single ray may lead to relative imbalance and transfer of load to an adjacent MTPJ. Even in experienced hands, the decision regarding whether to include the neighboring rays or not is difficult. The biggest limitation of the Weil osteotomy, however, is the tendency for joint stiffness and recurrent extension contracture to develop. Careful surgical technique (**Fig. 19**), including a double cut to elevate as well as translate the head fragment, and minimal soft tissue dissection,

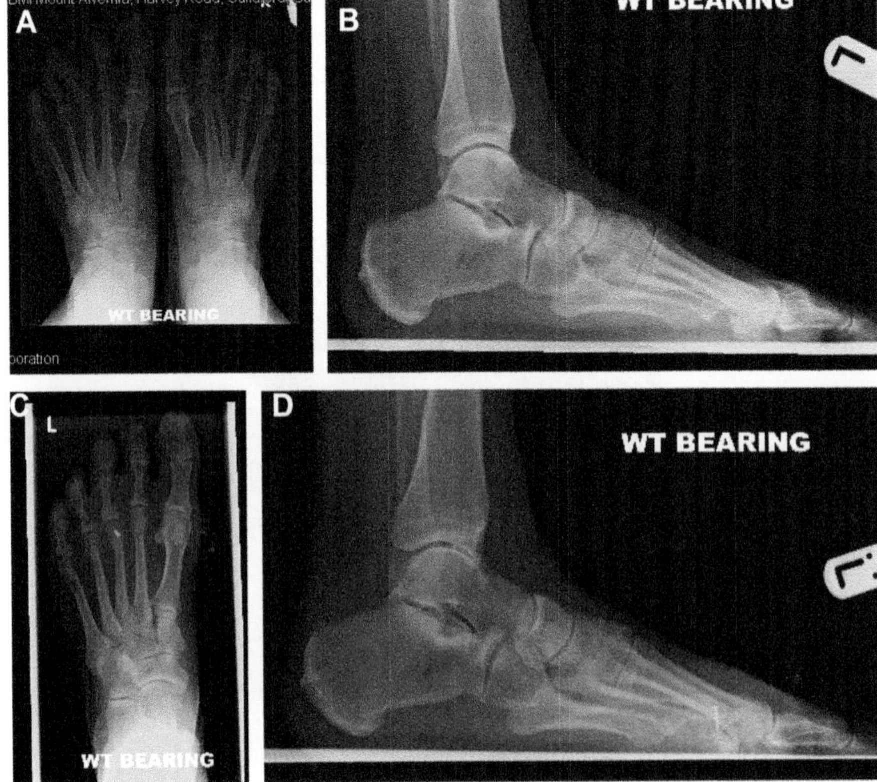

Fig. 20. (*A–D*) Weil and basal phalangeal osteotomies.

helps, but attention to postoperative splintage (in plantarflexion) and early plantarflexion stretching exercises are key.

Revision for the failed Weil osteotomy is challenging. Soft tissue release alone may suffice, but is best left until the scar tissue resulting from the first procedure is completely quiescent. This, in the authors' practice, means 12 months from the initial surgery. Barouk[14] describes a percutaneous release of all the dorsal structures. An open revision procedure allows more complete release, plantar release, and removal of fixation hardware. Any bony overgrowth at the osteotomy site can be dealt with as well.

Revision of the Weil osteotomy may be required to correct length, rotation, or depression of the head. Depending on the goals of the revision osteotomy, fixation may be difficult, not the least because of the existing screw hole in the metatarsal head. Potential solutions include use of a longer twist-off screw, conversion to a larger diameter Barouk or FRS screw, or use of K-wires.

Basal Metatarsal Osteotomy

Pain under a lesser MT (usually second) may complicate an otherwise successful Weil osteotomy. The MTP is flexible and reduced, but there is a prominence in the plantar surface of the foot and a discrete plantar callosity. The likely cause is plantar displacement of the MT head fragment at the time of the first Weil osteotomy. This inadvertent lowering can be avoided by means of a second horizontal cut when performing Weil osteotomies. Revision surgery at the site of original treatment may be needed if the MTPJ is stiff or extended. Consideration can be given instead to an extra-articular elevating osteotomy at the base of the MT. The BRT osteotomy is an excellent means of elevating a MT without subjecting the MTPJ to further soft tissue insult, and so minimizes the chance of MTPJ stiffness. Only a small closing wedge is required, because the distance from the MT head is relatively large. A small, angular correction proximally produces a large dorsal displacement of the head distally. The osteotomy is fixed with a compression screw and is intrinsically stable, allowing early mobilization.

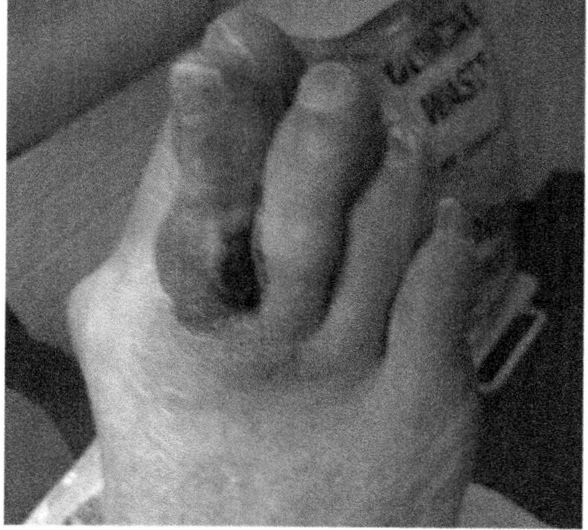

Fig. 21. Intractable infection.

Phalangeal Osteotomy

Closing wedge osteotomy of the base of the proximal phalanx is a useful means of indirectly correcting coronal plane deformity. Dissection is carried distally to the base of P1, where a (usually) medially based closing wedge is removed. The osteotomy is closed and held with an axial K-wire, often serving also to hold a PIP joint fusion or excision arthroplasty.[6] The closing wedge osteotomy can relieve abutment against an adjacent toe and is useful on occasion (**Fig. 20**).

Arthrodesis

Lesser MTPJ arthrodesis is an option as a salvage procedure for recalcitrant MTPJ pain, but is usually poorly tolerated by the patient. The authors have no personal experience with this procedure and do not recommend it.

Arthroplasty

Lesser MTPJ arthroplasty options include excision arthroplasty, interposition, and replacement. Excision arthroplasty experience in the rheumatoid population is very

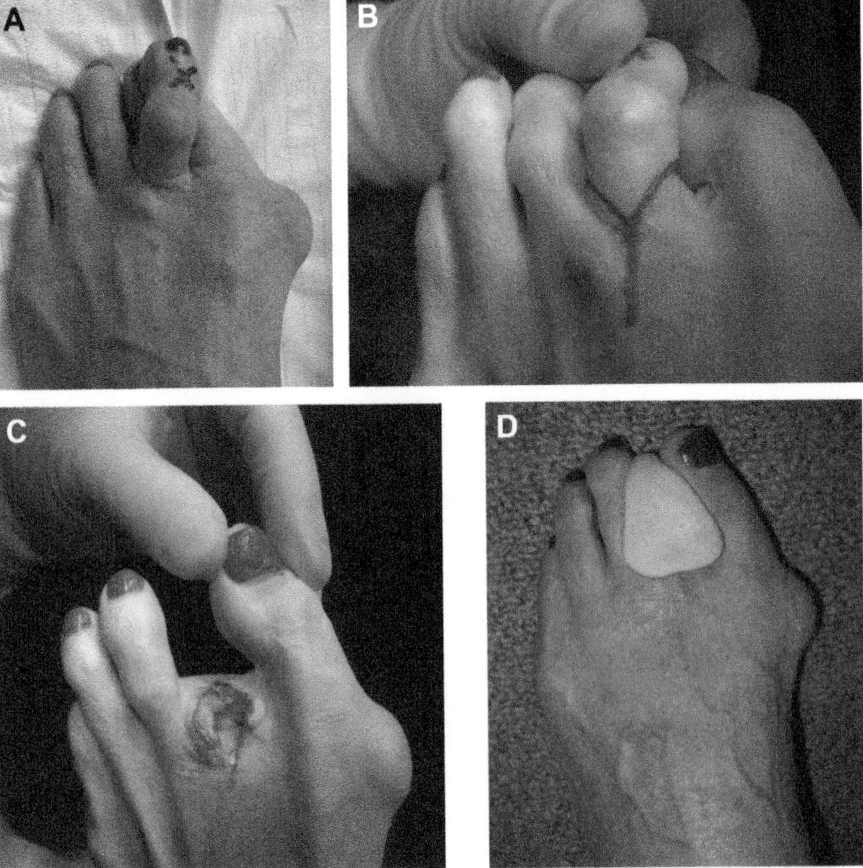

Fig. 22. (*A–D*) Toe amputation.

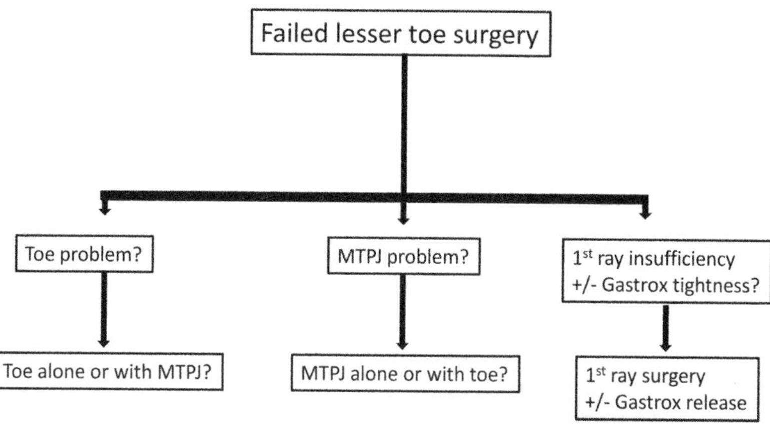

Fig. 23. Failed lesser toe surgery algorithm.

positive as part of a forefoot arthroplasty for end-stage disease[17,18]; treatment for an isolated lesser MTP problem in the patient not suffering from inflammatory arthropathy the indications are fewer. As mentioned, resection of the base of the proximal phalanx produces a short, stubby flail toe that is satisfactory in neither appearance

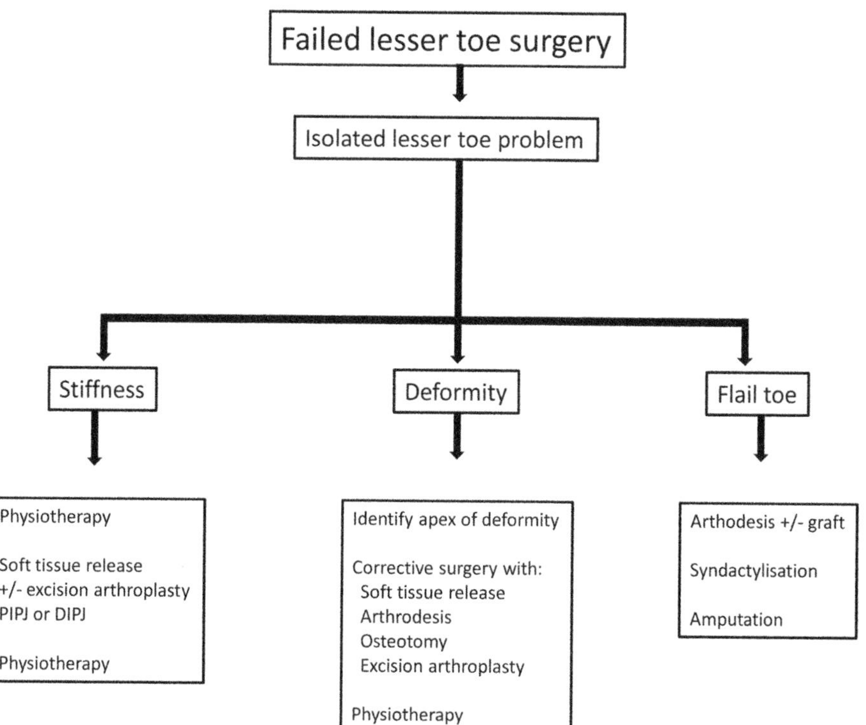

Fig. 24. Failed lesser toe algorithm - No MTP involvement.

nor function. Isolated lesser metatarsal head excision is likely to result in excessive load transfer to the neighboring MTPJ(s) with predictable consequences. It can be used in cases of end-stage arthritis of the MTPJ or in instances of fragmentation, nonunion, or osteonecrosis of the metatarsal head after prior osteotomy surgery. Use of dorsal capsular tissue, local tendon autograft, or allograft tendon can be interposed between the phalangeal base and metatarsal head remnant.

Replacement arthroplasty of the lesser MTPJs is fraught with potential complications, and there is little support in the literature for its use in revision situations. Anecdotally, a temporary button spacer is a useful means of preserving length if the MT head has to be removed. For all these reasons, interposition arthroplasty (Cobb 2 procedure) is the authors' preferred salvage option.

The Role of Amputation

Patients rarely request amputation, even of a chronically deformed painful lesser toe. The operation, however, has much to offer when the offending lesser toe is the source of severe pain, inability to wear conventional shoes, or intractable infection (**Fig. 21**).

The main problem with lesser toe amputation is the tendency for the adjacent toes to migrate toward each other. In the relatively immobile elderly patient, the use of an silicone gel or felt spacer can delay or prevent the development of secondary deformity and allow the use of off-the-shelf shoes.[7] The technique for amputation needs to be carried out expertly if the final result is to be cosmetically and functionally acceptable (**Fig. 22**). Amputation of all the lesser toes, known as the "Pobble" procedure (after Edward Lear's poem: "Everybody knows a Pobble has no toes") is no longer looked upon favorably. Instead, a more functional, balanced foot may be obtained with a transmetatarsal amputation, producing a durable, predictable result.

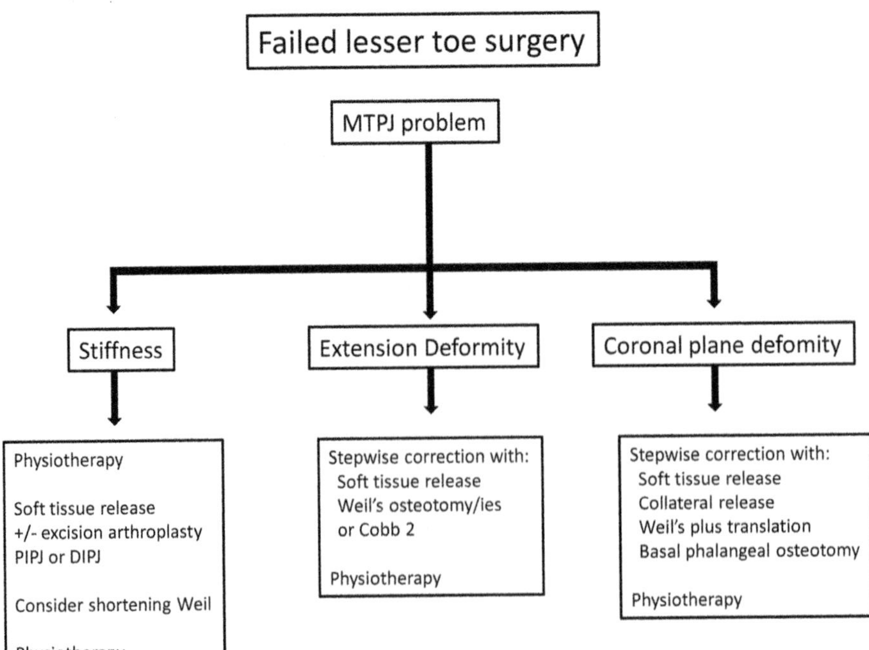

Fig. 25. Failed lesser toe algorithm - MTP joint involvement.

SUMMARY

Surgery of the lesser toes is a difficult balancing act, and revision procedures are challenging. It is vastly preferable that the correct procedure be chosen for the correct patient and performed properly from the outset. The flow charts below (**Figs. 23–25**) are not a rigid protocol, but rather the authors' personal algorithm, based on their own experience, which may help other surgeons facing a stiff, deformed or flail toe to make a reasoned decision.

REFERENCES

1. Coughlin MJ. Lesser toe abnormalities. Instr Course Lect 2003;52:421–44.
2. Myerson MS, Jung HG. The role of toe flexor-to-extensor transfer in correcting metatarsophalangeal joint instability of the second toe. Foot Ankle Int 2005;26:675–9.
3. Myerson MS, Filippi J. Interphalangeal joint lengthening arthrodesis for the treatment of the flail toe. Foot Ankle Int 2010;31:851–6.
4. Myerson MS, Filippi J. Bone block lengthening of the proximal interphalangeal joint for managing the floppy toe deformity. Foot Ankle Clin 2010;15:663–8.
5. Dhukaram V, Hossain S, Sampath J, et al. Correction of hammer toe with an extended release of the metatarsophalangeal joint. J Bone Joint Surg Br 2002;84:986–90.
6. Kilmartin TE, O'Kane C. Correction of valgus second toe by closing wedge osteotomy of the proximal phalanx. Foot Ankle Int 2007;28:1260–4.
7. Gallentine JW, DeOrio JK. Removal of the second toe for severe hammertoe deformity in elderly patients. Foot Ankle Int 2005;26:353–8.
8. Feeney S, Rees S, Tagoe M. Hemiphalangectomy and syndactylization for treatment of osteoarthritis and dislocation of the second metatarsal phalangeal joint: an outcome study. J Foot Ankle Surg 2006;45:82–90.
9. Conklin MJ, Smith RW. Treatment of the atypical lesser toe deformity with basal hemiphalangectomy. Foot Ankle Int 1994;15:585–94.
10. Haddad SL, Sabbagh RC, Resch S, et al. Results of flexor-to-extensor and extensor brevis tendon transfer for correction of the crossover second toe deformity. Foot Ankle Int 1999;20:781–8.
11. Bouche RT, Heit EJ. Combined plantar plate and hammertoe repair with flexor digitorum longus tendon transfer for chronic, severe sagittal plane instability of the lesser metatarsophalangeal joints: preliminary observations. J Foot Ankle Surg 2008; 47:125–37.
12. Lui TH. Arthroscopic-assisted correction of claw toe or overriding toe deformity: plantar plate tenodesis. Arch Orthop Trauma Surg 2007;127:823–6.
13. Lui TH, Chan LK, Chan KB. Modified plantar plate tenodesis for correction of claw toe deformity. Foot Ankle Int 2010;31:584–91.
14. Barouk LS. Scarf osteotomy for hallux valgus correction. Local anatomy, surgical technique, and combination with other forefoot procedures. Foot Ankle Clin 2000;5: 525–58.
15. Barouk LS. [Weil's metatarsal osteotomy in the treatment of metatarsalgia]. Orthopade 1996;25:338–44.
16. Trnka HJ, Nyska M, Parks BG, Myerson MS. Dorsiflexion contracture after the Weil osteotomy: results of cadaver study and three-dimensional analysis. Foot Ankle Int 2001;22:47–50.
17. Molloy AP, Myerson MS. Surgery of the lesser toes in rheumatoid arthritis: metatarsal head resection. Foot Ankle Clin 2007;12:417–33.
18. Mulcahy D, Daniels TR, Lau JT, et al. Rheumatoid forefoot deformity: a comparison study of 2 functional methods of reconstruction. J Rheumatol 2003;30:1440–50.

Freiberg's Disease

Rebecca A. Cerrato, MD

KEYWORDS

- Freiberg's disease • Osteochondrosis • Metatarsal
- Trauma • Circulatory disturbance

Originally described in 1914, Freiberg reported on a series of 6 cases with a similar "infarction" pattern of the second metatarsal head.[1] This pattern resulted in flattening and collapse of the head, with subsequent degenerative changes of the metatarsophalangeal (MTP) joint and ultimate arthritis in the final stages. Since then, numerous descriptions of the disease and opinions regarding its causes have been proposed. Although considered an uncommon occurrence, avascular necrosis of the second metatarsal is the fourth most common osteochondrosis.[2]

Broadly, osteochondroses are a family of disorders that result from an insult to the epiphysis that alters enchondral ossification and produces incongruity to the joint surface. Freiberg's disease is the only osteochondrosis more common in females, with a 5 to 1 female preponderance.[3] Both feet are involved equally. Typically only one lesion is found in a foot. Bilateral involvement is reported in less than 10% of cases.[4] The second metatarsal is affected in 68%, the third metatarsal in 27%, the fourth in 3%, and the fifth only rarely.[5] The peak age at onset for most osteochondroses is 11 to 17 years.

CAUSES

As with other osteochondroses, several potential explanations for Freiberg's disease exist. The two most popular theories include trauma and vascular compromise; however, many believe causes are multifactorial.[6–8] Moreover, other systemic disorders such as diabetes mellitus, systemic lupus erythematosus, and hypercoagulability have been implicated in the development of Freiberg's disease.[3,9]

Traumatic

Freiberg[1] in his original description documented a history of trauma in 4 of his 6 patients, suggesting a traumatic cause. Köehler[10] described the same condition in 1915 and argued against the role of trauma as the fundamental cause. In 1920, Freiberg acknowledged that simple trauma was not a "satisfying" explanation of the phenomenon.[11] Later, Smillie[12] supported the idea of a traumatic cause, noting that it was a function of repetitive dorsal trabecular stress injury. Smillie

Institute for Foot and Ankle Reconstruction, Mercy Medical Center, 301 St Paul Place, Baltimore, MD 21202, USA
E-mail address: rcerrato@mdmercy.com

Foot Ankle Clin N Am 16 (2011) 647–658
doi:10.1016/j.fcl.2011.08.008

argued that these events occur more frequently in feet with short, varus, or hypermobile first metatarsals.

The relative longer length of second metatarsal predisposes it to sustain greater stresses during normal gait.[8,13] The second metatarsal is the least mobile, thereby conferring the greatest stress at that metatarsal head distally. Hallux rigidus, hallux valgus, or any malalignment that disrupts the normal weight-bearing function of the first ray similarly increases the load assumed by the second metatarsal.[14] Helal and Gibb[6] injected silicone fluid into cadaveric MTP joints and studied the effects of passive range of movement. These investigators found that tense effusions produced incongruent movement, with a tendency for dorsal impingement on forced dorsiflexion.

Shoe wear has been argued to play a contributing role in the development of Freiberg's disease because of its predisposition in females. High-heeled shoes cause repetitive dorsiflexion forces across the MTP joints.[3] Multiple investigators have reviewed patients with known Freiberg and have not been able to directly link shoe wear with the disease.[7,8]

Vascular

Vascular deficiency has been attributed to necrosis of the metatarsal head. The second metatarsal is supplied by branches from the medial deep plantar artery and the dorsal metatarsal artery.[15] In 1981, Wiley and Thurston[16] performed injection studies on 6 cadavers and demonstrated that 2 of the 6 had absent second metatarsal arteries. Rather, they were supplied by collateral branches from the first and third metatarsals. The investigators assumed that a predisposing vascular pattern, in concurrence with an increased stress distribution, was the cause of avascular necrosis to the second metatarsal head.

Viladot and Viladot[17] noted that the blood supply to the metatarsal head comes from small vessels that penetrate the sides of the insertion of the joint capsule. Compression of these vessels from a joint effusion or swelling may compromise the blood flow.[3] The investigators further outlined the evolution of Freiberg's disease into five phases: (1) mechanical compression of the vessels, (2) arterial spasm, (3) epiphyseal ischemia, (4) occlusion of the vessels, and (5) formation of new blood supply from granulation tissue, bone resorption, remodeling, collapse, and subsequent joint arthrosis.

PATHOPHYSIOLOGY

Omer[18] described the pathologic origin of articular osteochondroses in three stages. In the first stage, intraarticular and periarticular soft tissues swell and engorge. The second stage exhibits irregularity of the epiphyseal contour. In the final stage, the necrotic tissue is gradually replaced.

Smillie[12] outlined the macroscopic progression of the disease into five stages.

Stage I: A narrow fissure fracture develops in the ischemic epiphysis. Surrounding cancellous bone appears sclerotic. When compared with adjacent metaphyseal bone, the epiphysis is deficient or devoid of blood flow.

Stage II: Absorption of cancellous bone occurs within the metatarsal head centrally, causing collapse of the overlying subchondral bone. The overlying cartilage is depressed, hinging on the intact cartilage at the plantar aspect, altering the contour of the articular surface.

Stage III: Further absorption occurs, allowing the central portion to sink deeper and leaving projections on either side. The plantar cartilage remains intact.

Stage IV: The central portion of the articular surface has sunk enough to fracture the plantar hinge. Peripheral projections have fractured to produce loose bodies. Restoration of the anatomy is no longer possible.

Stage V: The final stage demonstrates arthrosis with marked flattening. Only the plantar portion of the metatarsal cartilage retains the original contour. Most of the loose bodies have reduced in size and the shaft of the metatarsal is thickened and dense.

CLINICAL PRESENTATION

Patients frequently present with the complaint of pain localized to the involved metatarsal head region. They will often describe a sense that they are walking on something hard, such a stone or marble. Symptoms are exacerbated with walking, particularly barefoot.

On examination, the toe may have a swollen appearance that can range from mild fullness around the MTP joint to fusiform swelling of the affected toe (**Fig. 1**). Elevation of the toe may be present. In more chronic or advanced stages, sagittal or coronal plane malalignment may develop, such as hammer toes or crossover deformities. Range of motion across the MTP joint is variably reduced, with crepitation palpated. Along the plantar fat pad, a callus may develop under the involved metatarsal head. In earlier stages, tenderness over the metatarsal head or MTP joint may be the only physical sign.

Lachman testing evaluates joint instability and is graded based on the amount of translation of the proximal phalanx relative to the metatarsal head.[3,19] Comparison with the contralateral foot is necessary. The test is considered abnormal when the joint subluxes dorsally. This subluxation typically will reproduce the patient's pain.

IMAGING

Radiographs

Careful inspection of weight-bearing foot films often reveals subtle changes in early stages of the disease. The earliest finding is joint space widening, which can be present 3 to 6 weeks following onset of symptoms.[20] As the disease progresses, increased bone density within the subchondral bone and flattening of the metatarsal head may be seen (**Fig. 2**). With the ability to visualize the dorsum of the metatarsal

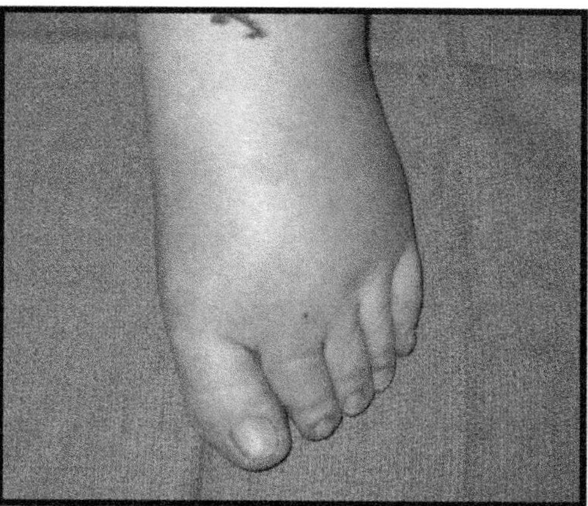

Fig. 1. Patient presented with complaints of pain under second metatarsal head with fusiform second toe swelling.

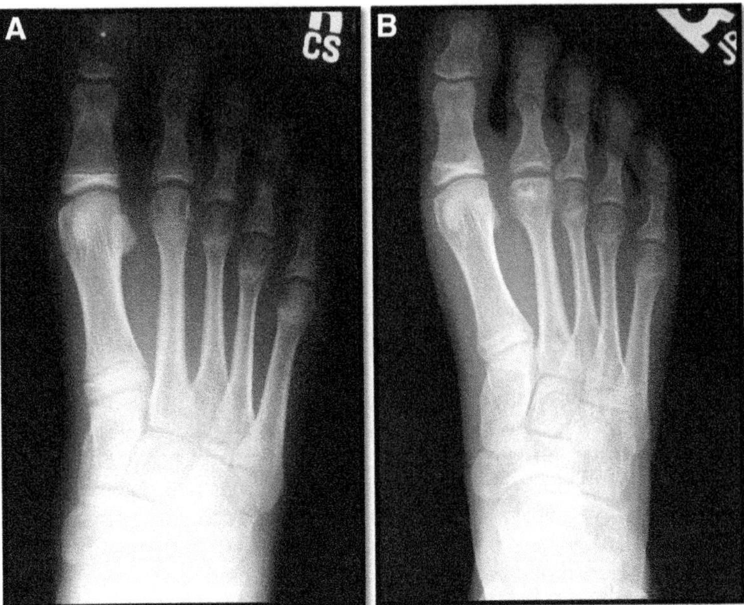

Fig. 2. (*A*) On initial evaluation, the patient's anteroposterior radiograph was unremarkable. (*B*) At follow-up one year later, flattening of the metatarsal head is easily apparent.

head, the oblique radiograph can be a valuable tool in demonstrating abnormalities otherwise unapparent on the anteroposterior view (**Fig. 3**).[21] Later radiographic findings include central joint depression, rarefaction, loose bodies, and sclerosis.[12] Thickening of the metatarsal shaft can be a late finding and may represent a response to abnormal stress.[7] The final stage of the process involves frank joint space narrowing and arthrosis.

Lee and colleagues[22] reviewed the radiographs of 72 normal feet. They noted that 10% of patients demonstrated bilateral flattened appearance to the second metatarsal head with joint space widening compared with adjacent joints. In the absence of increased subchondral bone density, the investigators argued that this may represent a normal anatomic variant.

Magnetic Resonance Imaging

Magnetic resonance imaging (MRI) of a painful metatarsal can assist in early detection of Freiberg's disease when undetectable on plain radiographs.[23] MRI images reflect changes within marrow intensity. Consistent with osteonecrosis seen elsewhere in the body, MRI may demonstrate hypointense signal on T1-weighted images and mixed hypointense and hyperintense signals on T2-weighted images. Flattening of the head is also noted on sagittal images.

Bone Scan

Early-stage disease may show a photopenic area surrounded by a very active revascularized collar, typical for the pattern of early avascular necrosis.[4] The photopenia was appreciated only on pinhole collimator images and predates any visible radiographic findings. The pinhole collimator is a conical collimator with a small

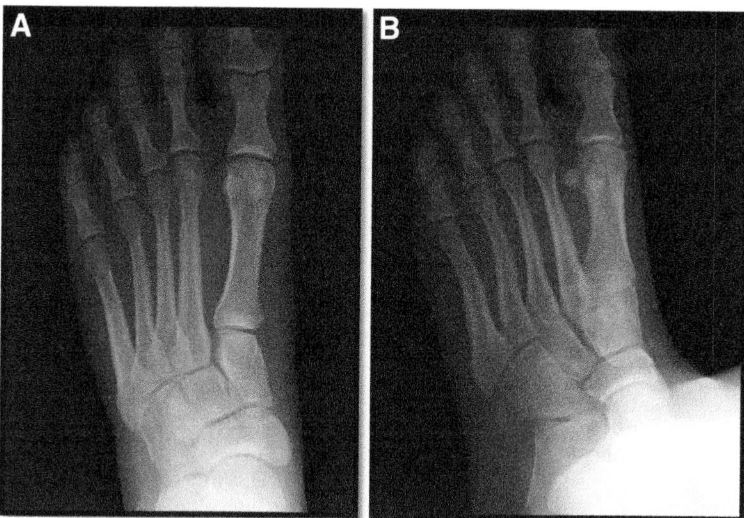

Fig. 3. (*A*) The anteroposterior radiograph demonstrates minimal flattening of the second metatarsal head. (*B*) The oblique radiograph reveals flattening of the dorsal metatarsal head.

circular aperture that produces an inverted image of an object. The image is magnified, optimizing resolution in the evaluation of circumscribed areas. In later stages, scintiscan imaging would reveal diffuse hyperactivity secondary to revascularization, repair, and ultimate arthritic involvement of the MTP joint.

STAGING

Different staging schemes have been suggested by various authors, correlating physical and radiographic findings. The Smillie classification was outlined earlier in the pathophysiology section. Gauthier and Elbaz[5] reported on the findings of 88 cases of Freiberg, creating a classification scheme with four types. The investigators separated the types by the degree of osteonecrosis and potential for subsequent healing, from stage 0 to stage IV. New vessel formation and consolidation can occur at any stage; however, permanent changes occur with the later stages. In stage 0, the earliest insult was a march fracture of the epiphysis. The disruption of blood flow results in osteonecrosis (stage I). Healing during both of these stages can maintain a normal joint. In stage II, the plantar isthmus of articular cartilage remains intact (**Fig. 4**). Consolidation at stage II results in a mildly flattened metatarsal head that may or may not be symptomatic. Restoration is possible because the blood supply remains intact and is unaffected by the ischemic process in the underlying bone. Stage III corresponds to Smillie's stage IV wherein the central portion and peripheral projections fracture, producing loose bodies. At this stage, damage is irreparable. Stage IV involves advanced degenerative arthrosis.

In 1987, Thompson and Hamilton[24] described a staging scheme according to the degree of the vascular insult and its appropriate treatment. Type I Freiberg's disease involves a transient lesion that heals spontaneously without loss of articular cartilage. Treatment requires only protection with reduced activity, low heels, and a metatarsal pad. Type II lesions represent a larger vascular insult with periarticular osteophytes; however, the articular cartilage is largely preserved. Treatment for this stage can be

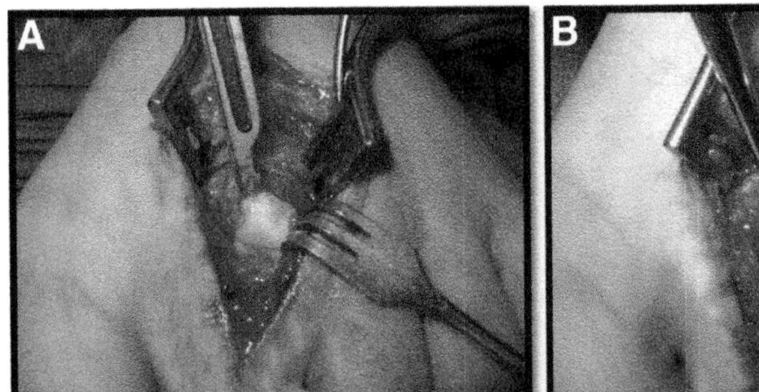

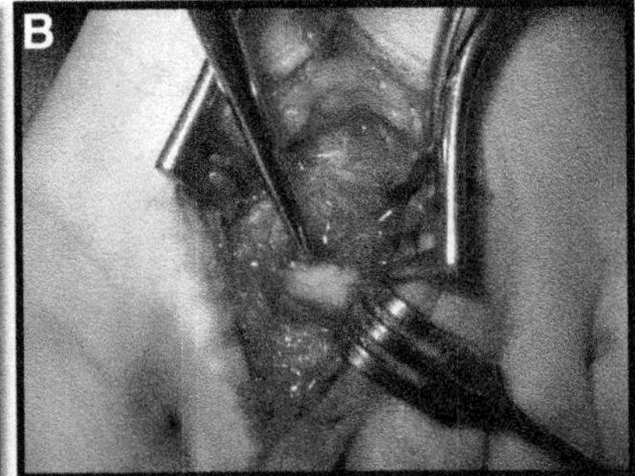

Fig. 4. (*A, B*) The plantar articular cartilage is intact in Gauthier and Elbaz's stage II disease.

limited to debridement of the spurs and synovectomy. Type III Freiberg's disease includes the most severe involvement marked by articular destruction and degenerative changes. Management of this stage involves a DuVries arthroplasty or interpositional arthroplasty. Type IV lesions are uncommon and involve multiple metatarsal heads, likely representing a form of epiphyseal dysplasia. Surgical treatment should be individualized based on the stage of lesion at each metatarsal head.

CONSERVATIVE MANAGEMENT

The goal of nonoperative management is not only to alleviate symptoms but to also minimize epiphyseal deformity. Activity modification, oral antiinflammatory medications, protected weight bearing, and shoe-wear modifications comprise the foundation for early treatment. Protected weight bearing can range from walking in a stiff-soled shoe, fracture boot, or cast to crutch use and non–weight bearing. Rocker-bottom soles with stiff semirigid material can provide relief during gait.[3] Orthoses with metatarsal bars are designed to offload the painful metatarsal head. Helal and Gibb[6] observed that the majority of Smillie stage I to III patients responded to these measures without long-term disability.

Morandi and colleagues[25] described a technique for skeletal traction using a metal arch that was supported by a below-knee cast. Patients were maintained in the device for 30 days. Patients reported significant decreases in pain within 42 days. Bisphosphonate therapy has also been studied in the treatment of femoral head osteonecrosis, with evidence supporting its use.[26] However, no research has been conducted to establish the efficacy and safety of bisphosphonate therapy for small joint osteochondrosis such as Freiberg's disease.

SURGICAL MANAGEMENT

A large number of surgical procedures have been proposed in the treatment of Freiberg's disease once conservative measures have failed. Freiberg[1] in his original report described removal of loose bodies presumably for later stages. Little consensus exists as to which type of surgical procedure should be done. In a review by Carmont and colleagues,[3] surgical options were divided into two basic categories. The first was procedures that attempt to alter the abnormal physiology and biomechanics that may predispose an individual to the disease. These alterations include core decompression and corrective osteotomies. The latter category involves procedures that restore articular congruency or address the arthritic sequelae encountered in the later stages. These procedures include debridement, osteotomy, grafting, and arthroplasty.

Core Decompression

Core decompression is intended to relieve the elevated intraosseous pressure at the site of avascular bone, allowing revascularization of the necrotic bone. Extensively studied in the hip, only two case reports involving core decompression for the metatarsal head have been described.[27,28] Patients from both studies had pain with no structural changes seen on plain radiographs. Decompression was performed using a 1.1-mm Kirschner wire to make multiple drill holes in the metatarsal head. Both case reports reported complete pain relief and no interval structural changes to the metatarsal head.

Open Joint Debridement

Joint debridement is a relatively simple procedure that can be applied at any stage of the disease. Removal of loose bodies, osteophytes, and delaminated cartilage has been recommended with reported good results.[1,6,7,12] Smillie emphasized joint debridement in a report outlining an osteotomy and graft procedure.[12] Helal and Gibb[6] modified Smillie's technique with the addition of a Kirschner wire across the joint and a short-leg cast for 6 weeks. Joint debridement is a simple, reproducible procedure that is not very destructive and does not prevent subsequent procedures (**Fig. 5**).

Arthroscopic Joint Debridement

Two reports discuss results of arthroscopic debridement of Freiberg's disease.[29,30] Maresca and colleagues[30] reported results on a single patient who underwent bilateral arthroscopic joint debridement and drilling at first metatarsal head. At 2 years following surgery the patient was without symptoms, and a follow-up MRI exhibited restructuring of the lesion. Carro and colleagues[29] reported results on a patient with Smillie stage IV disease who underwent arthroscopic joint debridement and resection of the base of the proximal phalanx. Similarly, at 2 years the patient was symptom-free.

Perichondral Grafting

Smillie[12] described cutting a 14-mm by 5-mm slot on the dorsum of the shaft across the epiphysis and metaphysis. At stages I and II, blood supply is reestablished by breaking down the sclerosis on either side of the fracture. With stage III, the fragment

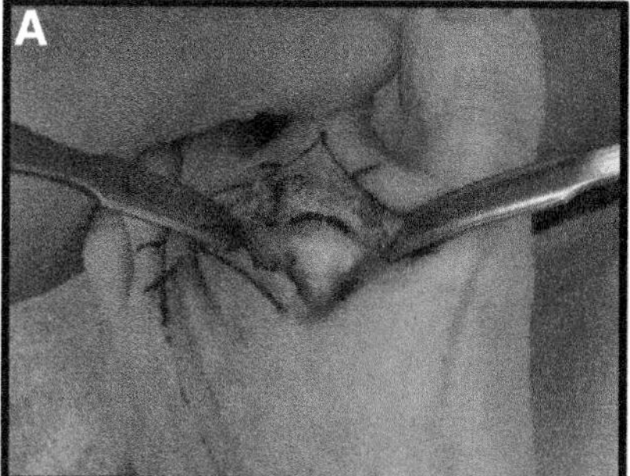

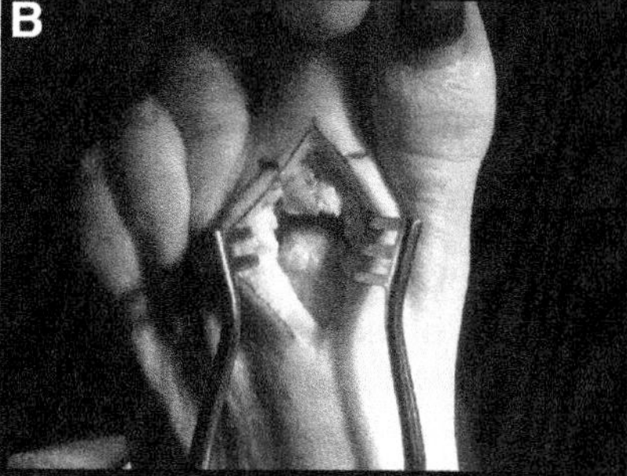

Fig. 5. (*A, B*) Open surgical debridement involves removal of loose bodies, peripheral osteophytes, and contouring of metatarsal head.

is gently levered on its hinge until the deformity is corrected. The resultant space is packed with autogenous bone graft. The epiphyseal plate is destroyed with multiple perforations. Helal and Gibb[6] reported on their experience with grafting. Of the 25 patients with Freiberg infraction, 11 patients were diagnosed with early disease (stage I or II) and suitable for grafting. At follow-up, 8 were clinically and radiographically normal, 1 was clinically normal, and 2 had pain with running and with wearing high-heeled shoes.

Osteochondral transplantation has been studied for its role in Freiberg's disease.[31–33] Hayashi and colleagues[32] were first to describe a case report of an osteochondral graft harvested from the femoral condyle to the metatarsal head. At 1 year follow-up, the patient returned to full activities with no pain. Later, other case reports and series have commented on similar results.[31,33]

Metatarsal Osteotomies

The two basic types of osteotomies are dorsiflexion and shortening. The objective for the dorsal closing wedge osteotomy is to redirect the plantar articular cartilage to articulate with the proximal phalanx (**Fig. 6**). The goal of the shortening osteotomy is to decompress or offload the abnormal metatarsal head.

In 1979, Gauthier and Elbaz[5] first described the dorsiflexion osteotomy of the metatarsal head in a series of 53 cases. The osteotomy was at the site of the lesion, using the healthy lower part of the metatarsal head to replace the necrotic bone. The investigators reported persistent symptoms in only 1 of their patients. In retrospective studies, Kinnard and Lirette[34,35] presented the results of 15 patients with an average 50-month follow-up. The procedure involved a wide arthrotomy, joint debridement, and removal of an intraarticular dorsal wedge of bone. Initially cerclage wires were used to secure the osteotomy; because of the development of secondary extensor tendinitis in some patients, the technique was modified to use absorbable suture. Average shortening of 2 to 5 mm occurred; however, the investigators noted that there were no cases of transfer metatarsalgia. In 2007, Capar and colleagues[36] reported results following debridement, synovectomy, and dorsal closing wedge osteotomy fixated with Kirschner wires. The investigators followed 19 patients an average of 44 months. The results were good to excellent in 84.2% of patients. Others have described the technique of using bioabsorbable pins for fixation while allowing early joint motion.[37] Arguments against the dorsiflexion osteotomy include technical difficulty, possible increased risk for avascular necrosis, and the potential to produce a transfer lesion.

Smith and colleagues[38] described a metatarsal shortening osteotomy procedure intended to offload the abnormal metatarsal head. The extraarticular osteotomy was performed at the metatarsal neck and stabilized with T-shaped small fragment plate. The investigators presented 16 cases with an average 4.9-year follow-up. Fifteen patients demonstrated pain relief within 12 months, and a postoperative pedobarograph study showed reduction in pressure over the affected metatarsal head. Seven patients had joint stiffness, and 4 of these had dorsiflexion contractures with toe elevation.

Excision/Interpositional Arthroplasty

In later stages of the disease, metatarsal head excision can eliminate joint pain and has been frequently used and discussed in the older literature.[6] Despite adequate pain relief, excision of the diseased metatarsal head can result in pressure metatarsalgia under adjacent lesser metatarsals, progressive hallux valgus, and shortening of the toe. Additionally, excision of the proximal phalanx base will destabilize the toe, again imbalancing the forces at the forefoot.[7]

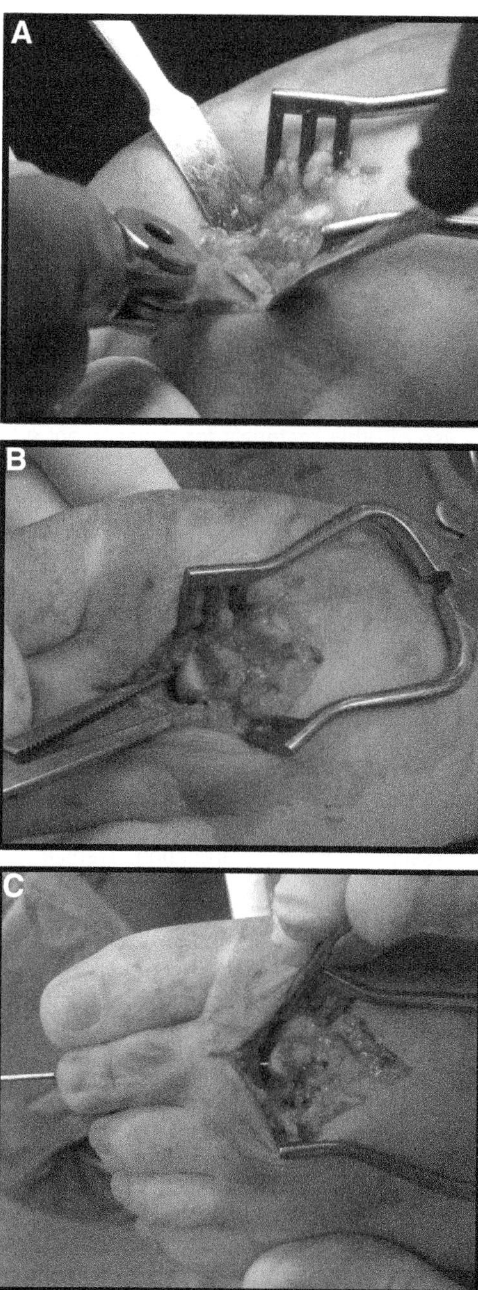

Fig. 6. (*A–C*) Dorsiflexion osteotomy performed to rotate healthier plantar articular cartilage of the second metatarsal head against proximal phalanx cartilage surface.

Interpositional arthroplasty using soft tissues have been widely used in the treatment of degenerative joint disease of the lesser MTP joints.[39] Tendon interposition can facilitate the maintenance of the apparent joint space and prevent bone impingement during motion. Tissues used include both flexor and extensor tendons.

Thompson and Hamilton[24] described treatment of type III lesions by creating a fibrous interposition by taking a purse-string suture in the volar plate and collateral ligaments. Additional tissues used include the dorsal capsule, extensor digitorum longus, extensor digitorum brevis, and peroneus longus free graft.[39–42]

Replacement Arthroplasty

Joint replacement arthroplasties have been created for the treatment of end-stage degenerative joint disease. Silicone implant arthroplasty has been described in the treatment of advanced Freiberg's disease.[6,43] Cracchiolo and colleagues[43] reported that in a series of 31 feet, 6 were surgically treated for advanced Freiberg's disease with a double-stemmed silicone implant in 5 and a single-stem condylar implant in 1. At 3-year follow-up, 4 patients reported good results and 2 had reservations. Potential complications include prosthetic failure, loosening, transfer metatarsalgia, synovitis with local bone resorption, and infection.

In recent years the use of other materials for replacement arthroplasty has been explored. A titanium hemiarthroplasty of the proximal phalanx combined with metatarsal head debridement was discussed in a case report.[44] Townshend and Greiss[45] reported on experience with total ceramic arthroplasty for the treatment of destructive disorders of the lesser MTP joints. In the case series, 6 patients received the implant as treatment for stage V Freiberg or failed previous surgery for Freiberg's disease. At 23 months, 8 reported good or excellent outcomes. Similar to silicone implants, these newer devices carry the potential for implant loosening, bone erosion, infection, and a stiff, floating toe.

COMPLICATIONS

Although joint debridement procedures do not prevent other surgical techniques, they do alter the anatomic conditions at the MTP joint, which can precipitate the condition further. Similarly, metatarsal osteotomies introduce the risk of disrupting the tenuous blood supply and can result in further deterioration. Transfer metatarsalgia, stress fracture, arthrofibrosis, and surgical wound infection are also potential complications following any surgical procedure. Most commonly discussed, transfer metatarsalgia can result with excessive elevation. Dreeban and colleagues[46] studied the radiographic and pedobarographic results after distal dorsal closing wedge osteotomy. These investigators noted the occurrence of transfer metatarsalgia in 3 of 4 cases where the osteotomy resulted in more than 4.5 mm of head elevation.

SUMMARY

Freiberg's disease is a relatively uncommon disorder of the metatarsal head. Although trauma and circulatory disturbances likely contribute major roles in its development, it is widely accepted that Freiberg's etiology is multifactorial. Conservative treatment, focused on offloading and relieving stress, is uniformly accepted as the appropriate initial management. Surgical management can broadly be categorized as procedures which attempt to correct the pathophysiology and halt its progression, and procedures which address the sequelae of later stage disease. Newer strategies, including osteochondral transplantation, attempt to restore the damage metatarsal cartilage with a viable osteochondral plug.

REFERENCES

1. Freiberg AH. Infraction of the second metatarsal bone, a typical injury. Surg Gynecol Obstet 1914;19:191–3.

2. Omer GE. Primary articular osteochondroses. Clin Orthop 1981;158:33.
3. Carmont MR, Rees RJ, Blundell CM. Current concepts review: Freiberg's disease. Foot Ankle Int 2009;30:167–76.
4. Mandell GA, Harcke HT. Scintigraphic manifestations of infarction of the second metatarsal (Freiberg's Disease). J Nucl Med 1987;28:249–51.
5. Gauthier G, Elbaz R. Freiberg's infraction: a subchondral bone fatigue fracture. A new surgical treatment. Clin Orthop Rel Res 1979;93:93–5.
6. Helal B, Gibb P. Freiberg's disease: A suggested pattern of management. Foot Ankle Int 1987;8:94–102.
7. Katcherian DA. Treatment of Freiberg's disease. Orthop Clin North Am 1994;25:81.
8. Stanley D, Betts RP, Rowley DI, et al. Assessment of etiologic factors in the development of Freiberg's disease. J Foot Surg 1990;29:444–7.
9. Nguyen VD, Keh RA, Daehler RW. Freiberg's disease in diabetes mellitus. Skeletal Radiol 1991;20:425–8.
10. Köehler A. Typical disease of the second metatarsophalangeal joint. AJR Am J Roentgenol 1923;10:705.
11. Freiberg AH. The so-called infraction of the second metatarsal bone. J Bone Joint Surg Br 1926;8:257–61.
12. Smillie IS. Treatment of Freiberg's infraction. Proc R Soc Med 1967;60:29–31.
13. Donahue SW, Sharkey NA. Strains in the metatarsals during stance phase of gait implications for stress fractures. J Bone Joint Surg Am 1999;81:1236–44.
14. McMaster MJ. The pathogenesis of hallux rigidus. J Bone Joint Surg Br 1978;60: 82–7.
15. Peterson WJ, Lankes JM, Paulsen F, et al. The arterial supply of the lesser metatarsal heads: a vascular injection study in human cadavers. Foot Ankle Int 2002;23:491–6.
16. Wiley JJ, Thurston P. Freiberg's disease. J Bone Joint Surg Br 1981;63:459.
17. Viladot A, Viladot A. Osteochondroses: aseptic necrosis of the foot. In: Jahss M, editor. Disorders of the foot and ankle. 2nd edition. Philadelphia: Saunders, 1991: 617–38.
18. Omer GE. Primary articular osteochondroses. Clin Orthop 1981;158:33.
19. Coughlin M. Lesser toe abnormalities. Instr Course Lect 2003;52:421–44.
20. Hill J, Jimenez LA, Langford JH. Osteochondritis dissecans treated by joint replacement. J Am Podiatry Assoc 1979;69:556–61.
21. Hoskinson J. Freiberg's disease: a review of long term results. Proc R Soc Med 1974;67:106–7.
22. Lee SK, Chung MS, Baek GH, et al. Treatment of Freiberg disease with intra-articular dorsal wedge osteotomy and absorbable pin fixation. Foot Ankle Int 2007;28:43–8.
23. Mifune Y, Matsumoto T, Mizumo T, et al. Idiopathic osteonecrosis of the second metatarsal head. Clin Imaging 2007;31:431–3.
24. Thompson FM, Hamilton WG. Problems of the second metatarsophalangeal joint. Orthopedics 1987:10:83–9.
25. Morandi A, Prina A, Verdoni F. Treatment of Kohler's second syndrome by continuous skeletal traction. Ital J Orthop Traumatol 1990;16:363–8.
26. Agarwala S, Jain D, Joshi VR, et al. Efficacy of alendronate, a bisphosphonate, in the treatment of AVN of the hip. A prospective open-label study. Rheumatology (Oxford) 2005;44:352–9.
27. Dolce M, Osher L, McEneaney P, et al. The use of surgical core decompression as treatment for avascular necrosis of the second and third metatarsal heads. The Foot 2006;17:162-2.
28. Fieberg AA, Fieberg RA. Core decompression as a novel approach treatment for early Freiberg's infraction of the second metatarsal head. Orthopedics 1995;18:1177–8.

29. Carro LP, Golano P, Farinas O, et al. Arthroscopic Keller technique for Freiberg disease. Arthroscopy 2004;20:60–3.
30. Maresca G, Adriani E, Falez F, et al. Arthroscopic treatment of bilateral Freiberg's infraction. Arthroscopy 1996;12:103–8.
31. DeVries JG, Amiot RA, Cummings P, et al. Freiberg's infraction of the second metatarsal treated with autologous osteochondral transplantation and external fixation. J Foot Ankle Surg 2008;47:565–70.
32. Hayashi K, Ochi M, Uchio Y, et al. New surgical technique for treating bilateral Freiberg's disease. Arthroscopy 2002;18:660–4.
33. Miyamoto W, Takao M, Uchio Y, et al. Late stage Freiberg disease treated by osteochondral plug transplantation: a case series. Foot Ankle Int 2008;29:950–5.
34. Kinnard P, Lirette R. Dorsiflexion osteotomy in Freiberg's disease. Foot Ankle Int 1989;9:226–31.
35. Kinnard P, Lirette R. Freiberg's disease and dorsiflexion osteotomy. J Bone Joint Surg Br 1991;73:864–5.
36. Capar B, Kutluay E, Mujde S. Dorsal closing-wedge osteotomy in the treatment of Freiberg's disease. Acta Orthop Traumatol Turc 2007;41:136–9.
37. Gong HS, Baek GH, Jung JM, et al. Fixation of dorsal wedge osteotomy for Freiberg's disease using bioabsorbable pins. Foot Ankle Int 2003;24:876–7.
38. Smith TWD, Stanley D, Rowley DI. Treatment of Freiberg's disease: a new operative technique. J Bone Joint Surg Br 1991;73:129–30.
39. Özkan Y, Öztürk A, Özdemir R, et al. Interpositional arthroplasty with extensor digitorum brevis tendon in Freiberg's disease: A new surgical technique. Foot Ankle Int 2008; 29;488–92.
40. El-Tayeby HM. Freiberg's infraction: a new surgical approach. J Foot Ankle Surg 1998;37:23–7.
41. Lavery LA, Harkless LB. The interpositional arthroplasty procedure in treatment of degenerative arthritis of the second metatarsophalangeal joint. J Foot Surg 1992;31: 590–4.
42. Zgonis T, Jolly GP, Kanuck DM. Interpositional free tendon graft for lesser metatarsophalangeal joint arthroplasty. J Foot Ankle Surg 2005;44:490–2.
43. Cracchiolo A, Kitaoka HB, Leventen EO. Silicone implant arthroplasty for second metatarsophalangeal joint disorders with and without hallux valgus. Foot Ankle Int 1988;9:10–8.
44. Shih AT, Quint RF, Armstrong DG, et al. Treatment of Freiberg's infarction with the titanium hemi-implant. J Am Pod Med Assoc 2004;4:9590–3.
45. Townshend DN, Greiss ME. Total ceramic arthroplasty for painful destructive disorders of the lesser metatarso-phalangeal joints. The Foot 2006;17:73.
46. Dreeban S, Noble P, Hammerman S, et al. Metatarsal osteotomy for primary metatarsalgia: radiographic and pedobarographic study. Foot Ankle Int 1989;9:214–8.

Congenital Lesser Toe Abnormalities

Ho-Seong Lee, MD[a], Woo-Chun Lee, MD[b,*]

KEYWORDS

- Congenital deformity • Polydactyly • Macrodactyly
- Brachymetatarsia • Lesser toe • Foot

Congenital deformities of the lesser toes are relatively uncommon, but when present can prove challenging to the clinician. Congenital lesser toe deformities may not cause significant pain or functional problems, but often cause patient anxiety over their appearance. Marked enlargement or deviation of lesser toes can cause problems with shoe wear or painful impingement of the digits. Nonoperative care focuses on the use of wide toe box footwear to provide sufficient space for the digits. In cases with transfer metatarsalgia, a prescription orthotic insole with a cushioned forefoot and a metatarsal pad may relieve pressure. Surgical treatment is performed in some cases for cosmetic reasons, but more often is recommended to alleviate painful symptoms or shoe wear difficulties. In this article, polydactyly (including polysyndactyly) is reviewed in the first section, followed by a discussion of syndactyly, brachymetatarsia, and macrodactyly. Various operative treatments are presented.

POLYDACTYLY

Polydactyly of the foot is a congenital deformity presenting as supernumerary digits. The duplication may range from a fully formed, articulated osseous digit to a rudimentary soft tissue appendage, and may be accompanied by abnormalities of the associated metatarsal. Polydactyly of the foot can occur as an isolated disorder or as a part of a syndrome. Many children with polydactyly of the foot have associated abnormalities of the hand and other anomalies such as syndactyly and clinodactyly.[1] Polydactyly of the foot typically has little functional significance other than difficulty in shoe wearing.

Complete or incomplete syndactyly between the duplicated toes can be classified as polysyndactyly.[2] Both polydactyly and polysyndactyly have been classified under

---

The authors have nothing to disclose.
[a] Department of Orthopaedic Surgery, Asan Medical Center, College of Medicine, Ulsan University, 388-1 Pungnap-dong, Songpa-gu, Seoul 138-736, South Korea
[b] Department of Orthopaedic Surgery, Seoul Paik Hospital, College of Medicine, Inje University, 85, Jeo-dong, 2-ga, Jung-gu, Seoul 100-032, South Korea
* Corresponding author.
E-mail address: wclee@seoulpaik.ac.kr

Foot Ankle Clin N Am 16 (2011) 659–678
doi:10.1016/j.fcl.2011.08.011
1083-7515/11/$ – see front matter

the term polydactyly[3,4] because there are more than 5 toes. Because the accessory toes originate anywhere from the metatarsal to middle phalanx,[5] it may be more appropriate to use the terms polydactyly to include polysyndactyly, rather than differentiating between the two.

Incidence

The incidence is higher in Blacks (3.6–13.9 cases per 1000 live births) than in Whites (0.3–1.3 cases per 1000 live births).[6] In contrast to polydactyly of the hand, postaxial polydactyly is more common in the foot (80%), followed by preaxial polydactyly and then central polydactyly.[6] The central ray polydactyly has been found in 3% to 6%[1,7,8] and the preaxial polydactyly in 10.9% to 16% of cases in the foot.[1,9] In most cases, it occurs as an isolated trait with an autosomal-dominant inheritance pattern and variable expressivity.[10]

Classification

Polydactyly was initially subdivided into 3 groups according to the Temtamy and McKusic classification[10]: Preaxial polydactyly, referring to the duplication of the hallux; postaxial polydactyly, referring to the duplication of the fifth ray; and central ray duplication of the second, third, or fourth toes. This classification is commonly used for both hand and foot polydactyly; however, it does not differentiate the site of origin of the extra digit, which is important in planning surgery. A morphologic classification based on the anatomic configuration of the metatarsal was described by Venn-Watson[11]; however, many polydactylies that originate distally cannot be categorized by this classification.

Classification according to radiographic findings is inadequate in describing the characteristics of polydactyly in younger children in whom there is no osseous structure visible on radiographs yet. Classification by Watanabe and colleagues[1] based on ray involvement and the level of duplication is comprehensive, but very complicated.

Postaxial polydactyly

The postaxial polydactyly is more difficult to classify than preaxial or central polydactyly. Nogami[2] focused on fifth-toe polydactyly and described surgical treatment options. Lee and associates[12] suggested a classification system based on gross morphologic, radiographic, and operative findings. This classification system is helpful in determining the surgical plan because it classifies according to the site of origin of the extra digit as well as the potential for future bone growth. Postaxial polydactyly was classified according to the origin of the accessory digit as follows: Floating type, middle phalangeal (MP) type, proximal phalangeal type, fifth metatarsal type, or fourth metatarsal type. The floating type (**Fig. 1**) refers to the pedunculated nonarticulated accessory digit, similar to a rudimentary soft tissue tag or with a small osseous element, originating around the metatarsophalangeal joint. In the MP type (**Fig. 2**), there is complete syndactyly between the fifth and sixth toes.

The proximal phalangeal type is further divided into 3 subtypes according to the location of the extra digit: Proximal phalangeal lateral (PPL) type, proximal phalangeal medial (PPM) type, and proximal phalangeal head (PPH) type. The PPH type is similar to the MP type, but the accessory digit originates as a chondroma like appearance of the PPH and syndactyly (**Fig. 3**). The extra digit has a hypoplastic radiographic appearance in PPM type (**Fig. 4**). In the PPL type (**Fig. 5**), there is no syndactyly between duplicated toes, which have nearly the same size and shape and share the

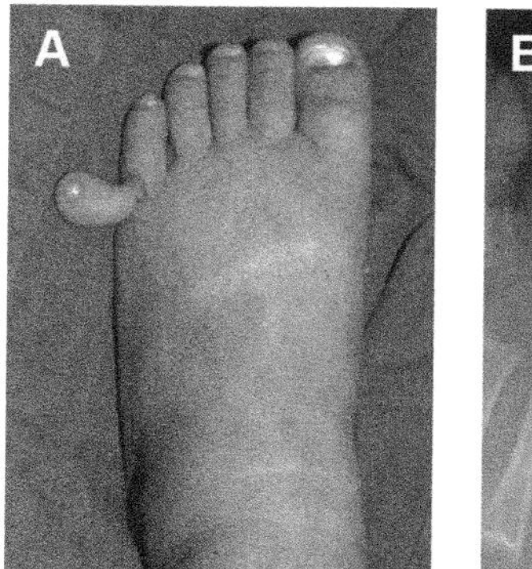

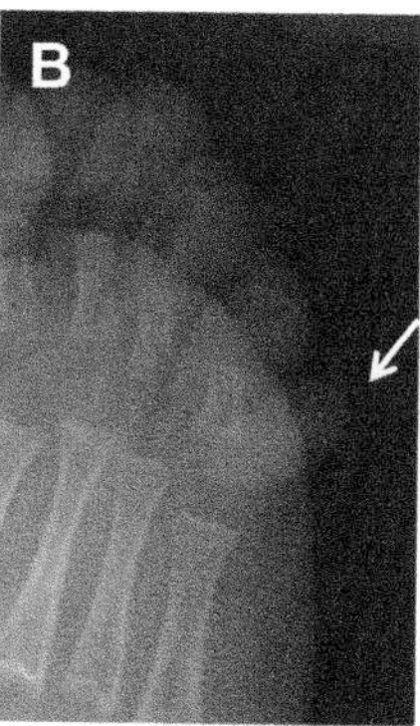

Fig. 1. Floating type. *A*, Preoperative photograph showing the pedunculated accessory digit similar to a rudimentary soft tissue tag. *B*, Anteroposterior radiographs showing the soft-tissue shadow originating from metatarsophalangeal joint (*white arrow*).

metatarsophalangeal joint. The PPL type is similar to metatarsal originated fifth MT type, but the fifth metatarsal bone has normal morphology.

In the fifth metatarsal type (**Fig. 6**), the lateral duplicated toe is abnormal and it is completely separated from the fifth toe. The supernumerary metatarsal bone arose from the fifth metatarsal shaft or had a duplicated symmetrical head and 2 articular surfaces.[11]

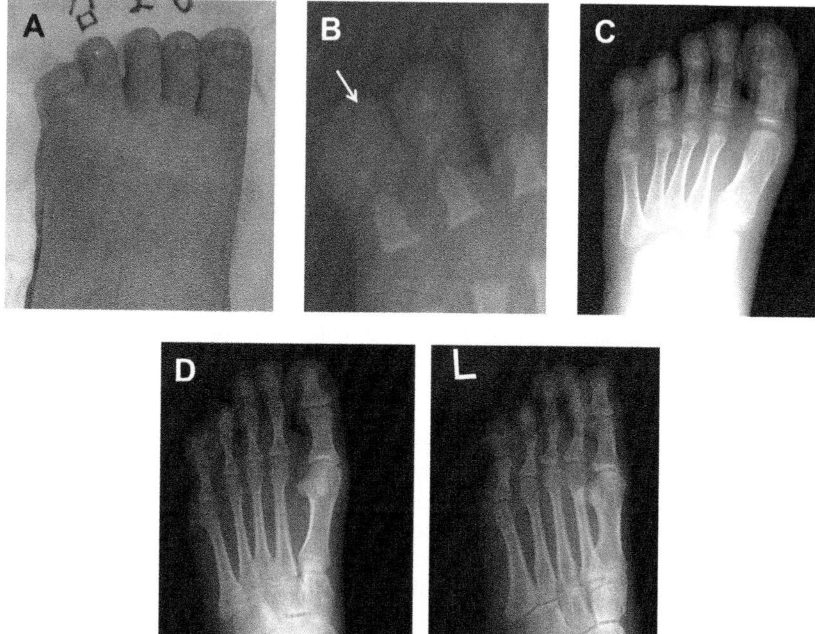

Fig. 2. MP type. *A*, Preoperative photograph showing complete syndactyly of fifth web and partial syndactyly of fourth web. *B*, Anteroposterior radiographs showing the medial accessory fifth toe at 1 year (*white arrow*). *C*, At 7 and 10 years. *D*, At 20 years.

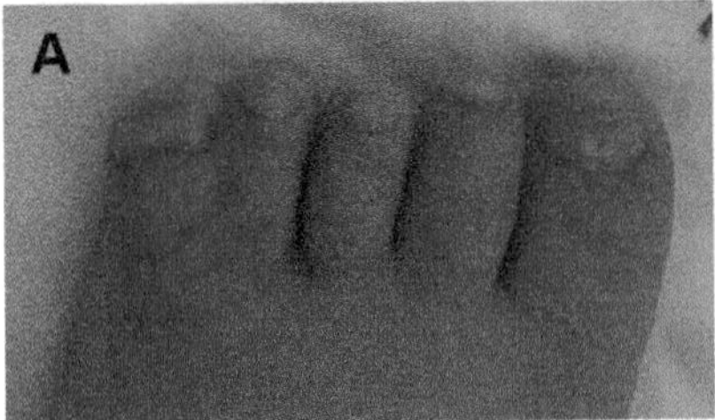

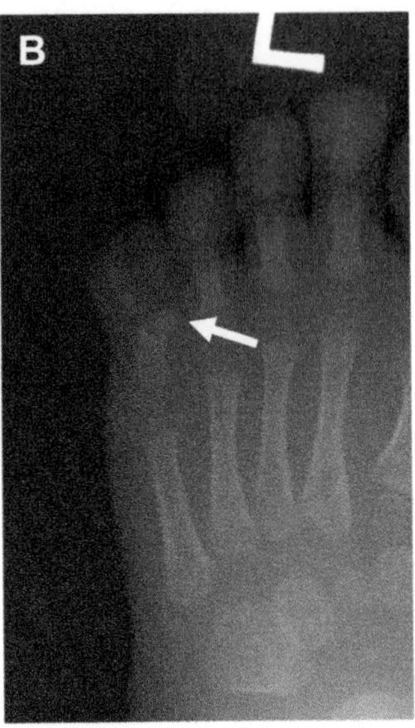

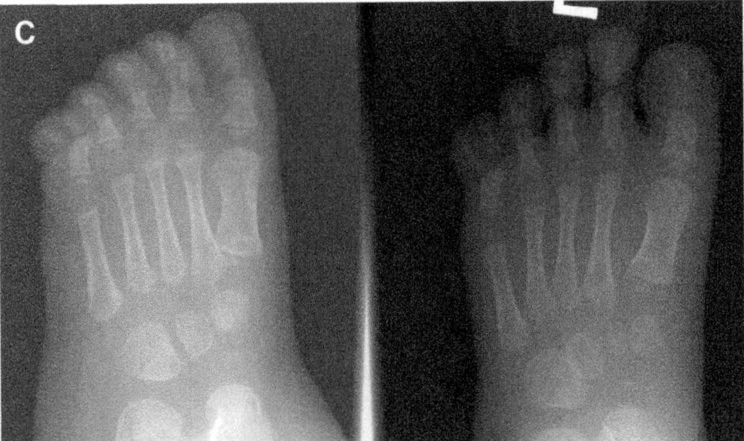

Fig. 3. PPH type. *A*, Anteroposterior radiographs showing the medial accessory digit similar to a chondroma in the phalangeal head region at 2 years. *B*, At 6 years (*white arrow*). *C*, At 6 years.

In the fourth metatarsal type (**Fig. 7**), the accessory digit originating from the fourth metatarsal has an abnormal appearance with syndactyly with the fifth digit in various patterns.

The extent of osseous fusion between duplicated toes and neighboring normal toes seems to be more severe when the accessory toes are more distal in origin. Also, growth retardation may occur with syndactyly. Duplications were bilateral in 19% and unilateral in 81% of patients.[12] In the bilateral duplications, symmetric abnormalities occurred in the 67% and the rest had different types in the 33%. The most common type in postaxial polydactyly was MP type.[12]

The optimal timing of the surgery for pedal polydactyly is controversial. Advantages of early surgery include better potential for soft tissue healing and bony remodeling. Most surgeons, however, delay the surgery until the patient is at least 1 year old to

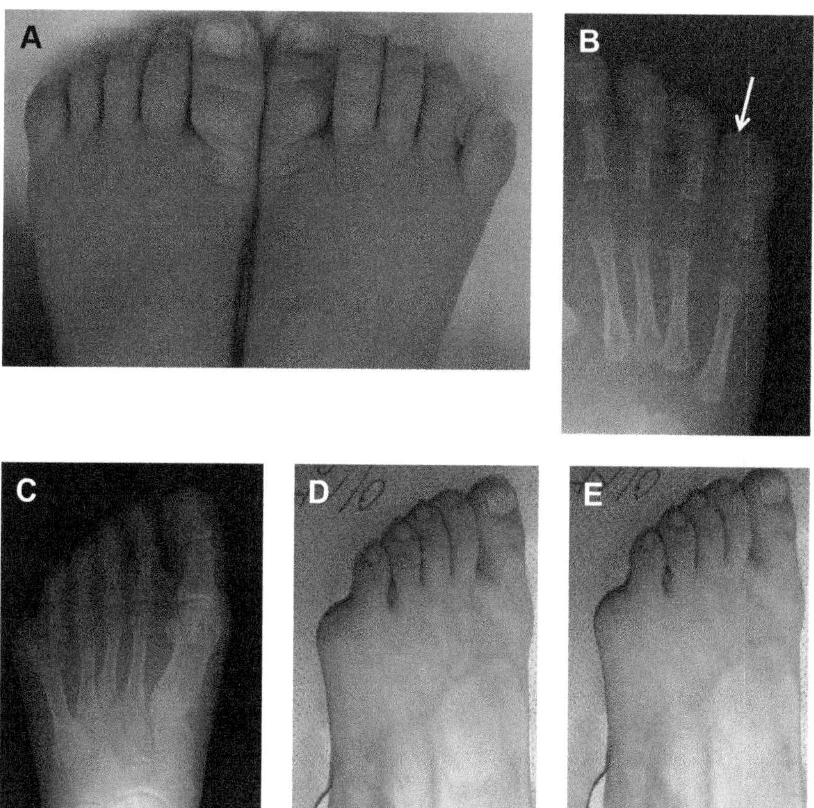

Fig. 4. PPM type. *A*, Preoperative photograph showing complete syndactyly of fifth web and no syndactyly of fourth web. *B*, Anteroposterior radiographs showing the medial hypoplastic accessory toe at 2 years (*white arrow*). *C*, At 5 years. *D*, After excision of the lateral 6th toe, the remained medial toe shows abnormal development at 22 years. *E*, Remained medial toe should have been excised in this case.

avoid potential problems with anesthesia and for better identification of the osseous and soft tissue structures. However, radiographs taken at 1 year often show a delay in appearance of the primary ossification centers of the hypoplastic phalanges.[13] This may make it difficult to distinguish which digit is the abnormal, duplicated toe. After additional bony growth, it is easier to radiographically distinguish a duplicated toe from a normal toe. Although surgeons may prefer delaying surgery, this waiting period may cause distress to the parents of these infants. The optimal time for surgery may therefore be when the patient is 2 to 4 years old. Earlier surgery is also recommended for individuals with preaxial type, particularly if it can cause difficulties in shoe fitting. Earlier excision is also recommended for a floating type extra digit, which is easily recognized. In patients who have metatarsal bowing or a shortened toe, the extra digit can be excised in stages; the first surgery occurs between 1 and 3 years old, with the second stage consisting of correction of any residual bony deformity after the completion of bone growth.

Excision of the outermost toe is recommended for the treatment of postaxial polydactyly, especially for the metatarsal type. It is not easy to treat the more distally

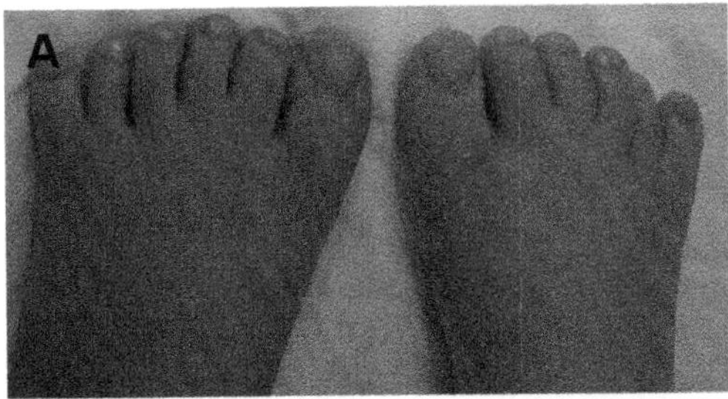

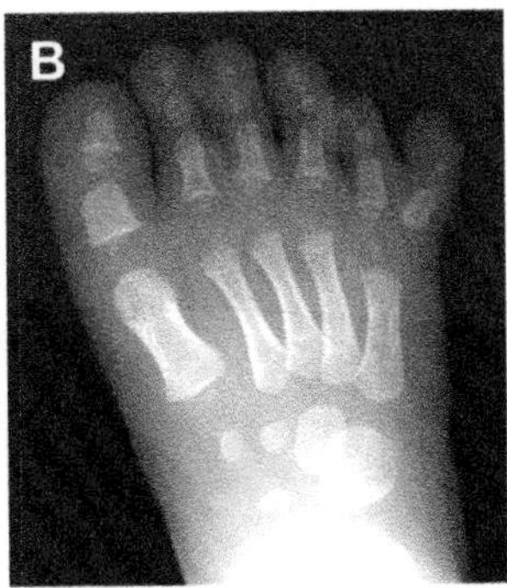

Fig. 5. PPL type. *A,* Preoperative photograph showing no syndactyly of fourth and fifth web, and symmetric medial and lateral toes. *B,* Anteroposterior radiographs showing the lateral accessory sixth toe at 4 years.

originated polydactyly. In postaxial MP type, the medial digit is an abnormally duplicated digit and should be excised.[1,12] When the inner duplicated toe is excised, webplasty can be performed using the remaining soft tissue to produce a better concealed, aesthetically pleasing scar. Complete excision of the duplicated digit, including the cartilage portion, is important; otherwise, polydactyly may recur later.

According to the Lee's classification,[12] the medial accessory fifth digit should be excised in the MP, PPH, PPM, and fourth metatarsal types. In the PPL, floating and fifth metatarsal types, the lateral accessory sixth digit should be excised.

We prefer to close the soft-tissue defect using the remaining skin after the excision of the accessory toe. However, in case of distally originated polydactyly, forceful approximation of the soft tissue defect after excision of the accessory digit may lead to skin necrosis, rotation deformity, or flexion contracture of the digits. A full-thickness skin graft is needed depending on the extent of syndactyly between the fourth and fifth toes. The extent of syndactyly between the fourth and fifth toes seemed to be more severe when the accessory toes had a more distal origin, and in the feet in which the extent of the syndactyly was more than one half, a full-thickness skin graft on the lateral side of the fourth digit is recommended rather than primary closure.

The main surgical steps for more distally originated polydactyly consists of excision of inner accessory digit, construction of an interdigital web using dorsal flap, primary repair of the inner wall defect of the fifth toe using a plantar skin flap, and covering the lateral wall of fourth toe using a full-thickness skin graft instead of primary repair.

Reconstruction of the deep transverse metatarsal ligament or collateral ligament, may be more difficult for children younger than 3 years old,[1] suggesting that, for these younger children, soft-tissue balancing is more important than ligament reconstruction. Moreover, there is no need for internal fixation using Kirschner wire, if soft tissues can maintain joint stability.

Preaxial polydactyly

Preaxial polydactyly has been found in 10.9% to 16% of cases of polydactyly of the foot.[1,9] Watanabe and co-workers[1] classified 36 preaxial polydactyly into 5 types according to duplication level: Tarsal type, metatarsal type, proximal phalangeal type,

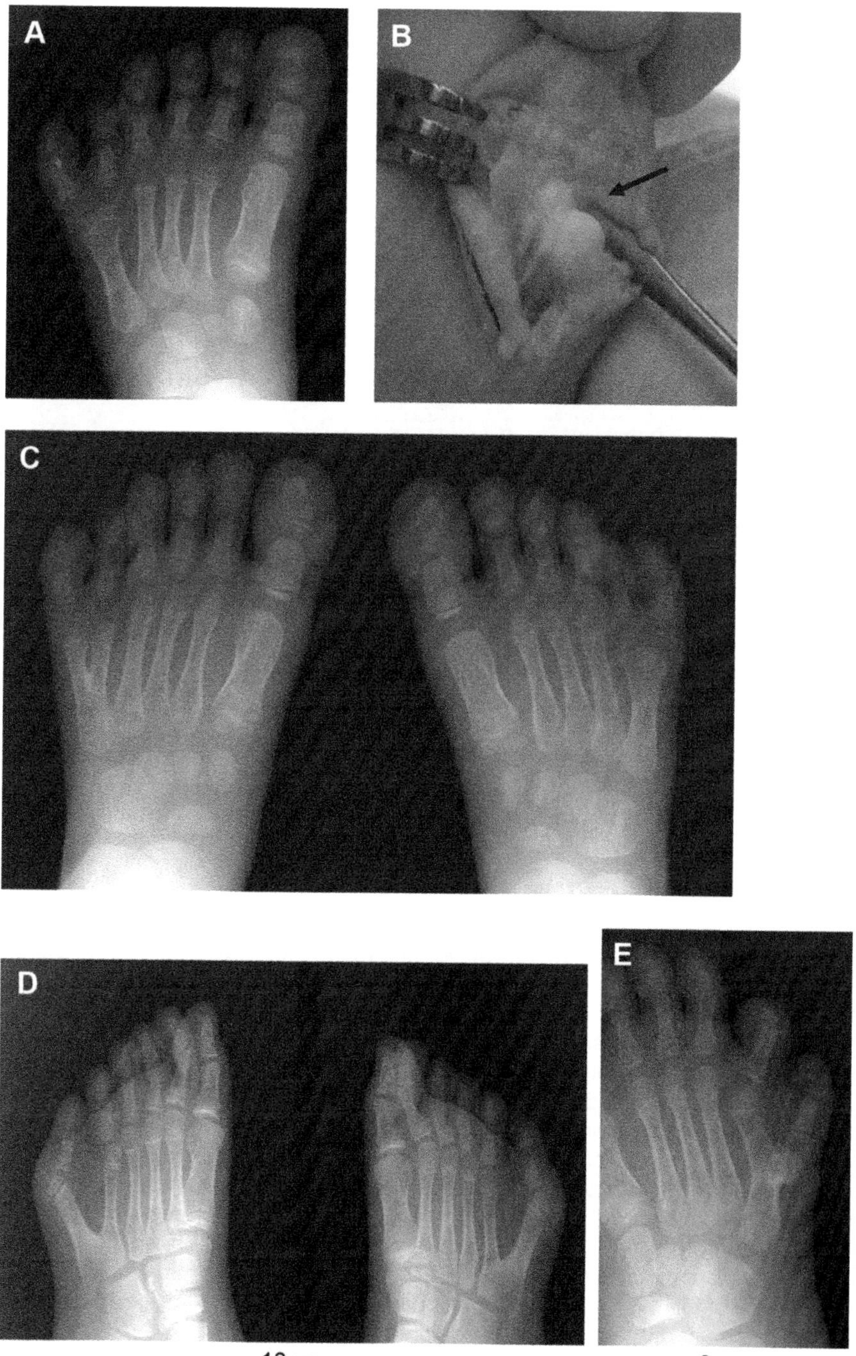

Fig. 6. Fifth metatarsal type. *A*, Preoperative anteroposterior radiograph. *B*, Intraoperative photograph showing the duplicated symmetrical fifth metatarsal head (*black arrow*). *B*, Anteroposterior radiograph showing the bowing of the fifth metatarsal bone and the accessory metatarsal bone arising from the metatarsal shaft. *D*, At 13 years old. *E*, At 8 years old.

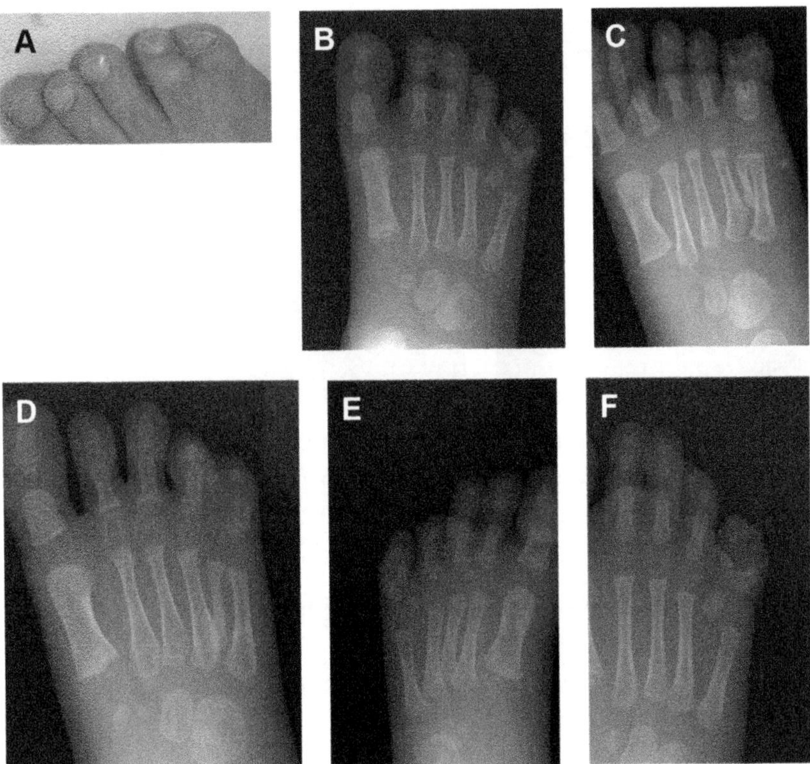

Fig. 7. Fourth metatarsal type. *A*, Preoperative photograph showing complete syndactyly of 5th web. *B–F*, Anteroposterior radiograph showing the accessory digit originating from the fourth metatarsal bone.

distal phalangeal type and floating type. Among them, the metatarsal type (13/36) and proximal phalangeal type (13/36) were most common; the tarsal type (1/36) was rarest. Morley and Smith[5] reported 5 preaxial types with similar pattern: 3 cases of metatarsal type and 2 cases of proximal phalangeal type. Masada and colleagues[9] classified 14 preaxial polydactyly into 4 types by modification of Venn-Watson classification: Ray duplication (2/14), completely duplicated phalanges (4/14), incompletely duplicated phalanges (6/14), and incompletely duplicated metatarsals (2/14).

Treatment of preaxial polydactyly is difficult. First, reattachment of the adductor hallucis tendon is mandatory to prevent hallux varus deformity after excision of the lateral accessory toe. Furthermore, congenital hallux varus deformity can be present with preaxial polydactyly (**Fig. 8**). Masada and colleagues[9] reported that 3 of 14 preaxial polydactyly deformities also had congenital hallux varus. Excision of the smaller rudimentary digit is preferred, with careful attention to soft tissue balancing to prevent deformity of the main hallux postoperatively.

Central ray polydactyly

The central ray polydactyly has been found in 3% to 6% of all cases of pedal polydactyly.[1,7,8] According to Watanabe and associates,[1] 16 central polydactyly were classified into 4 types according to duplication level: Metatarsal type, proximal

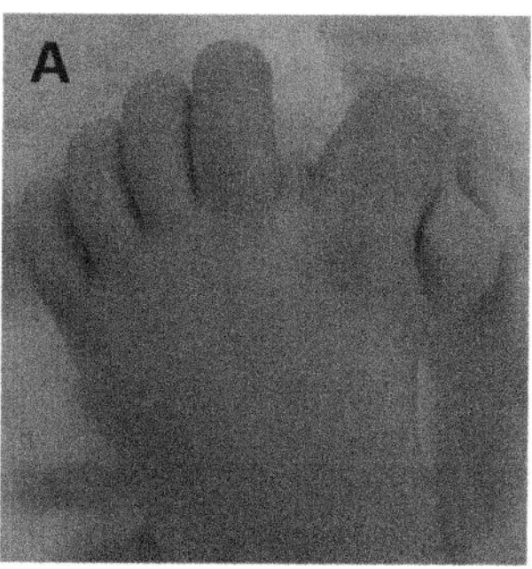

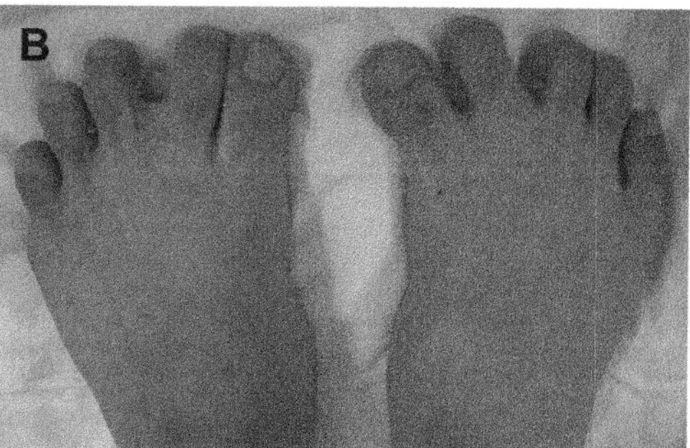

Fig. 8. Preaxial polydactyly with hallux varus deformity. *A*, Congential hallux varus deformity of at age 2. *B*, Postoperative hallux varus deformity of a 14-year-old patient.

phalangeal type, MP type, and distal phalangeal type. Fifteen of 16 central polydactyly were duplications of the second toe; distal the phalangeal type (6/16) was most common.

Little is known about the treatment of central ray polydactyly because of its rarity. Second toe duplication is most common, with both bone and soft tissue structures underdeveloped[1] (**Fig. 9**). In most cases, the extra digit can be excised through a racquet-shaped dorsal incision. Resection of the multiple extra toes in patients with central polydactyly creates a wide gap, which can be closed by repair of the transverse metatarsal ligament.[6,7]

Complications

After the removal of an inner digit, a transient abduction deformity may develop in the outer toe. The continuous adduction force of shoes gradually improve this deformity, however. Skin necrosis may occur after medial digit excision with webplasty for polysyndactyly. All, however, recovered spontaneously with simple moist dressings in 3 or 4 weeks without additional skin grafting.[11] In patients with the fifth MT type of polydactyly, medial bowing of the metatarsal bone was observed postoperatively. Hallux varus deformity can occur after excision of the lateral accessory toe in the preaxial type.

SYNDACTYLY

Syndactyly is defined as the persistence of webbing between adjacent digits. Toe syndactyly does not cause functional disability, as in the hand. Toe syndactyly affects

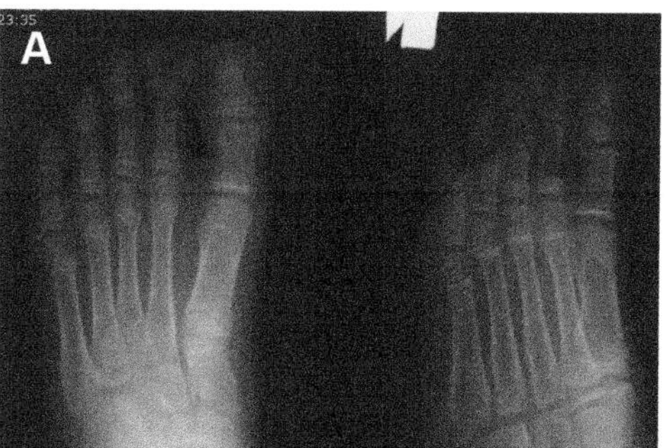

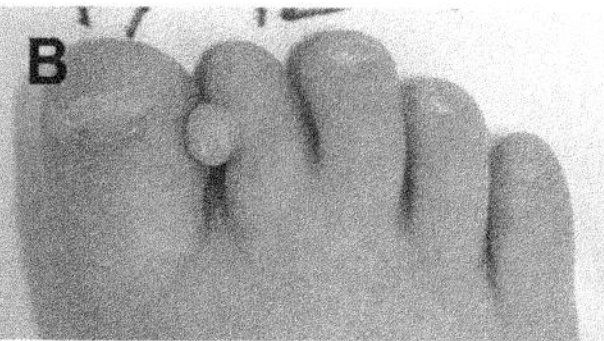

Fig. 9. Central ray polydactyly. *A*, Phalangeal duplication. *B*, Rudimentary type.

around 1/2000 people and occurs most commonly between the second and third toes.[14,15] The disorder is classified as "complete" if there is no web space at all and "partial or incomplete" if the connecting web extends partially between the toes. Congenital syndactyly may be inherited or occur as a developmental defect of the sixth and eighth weeks of fetal development.[16] Normally, the development of the web space between the second and third toes occurs last, which may explain the increased tendency for syndactyly to occur in that area.[14,15]

There are many associated anomalies with syndactyly such as Apert syndrome, Down syndrome, Adams–Oliver syndrome,[17] Pfeiffer syndrome,[18] scalp-ear-nipple syndrome,[19] nevus comedonicus syndrome,[20] and Kindler syndrome.[21]

Treatment

The goal of syndactyly surgery is to restore normal anatomy, minimize associated morbidity, and limit the-long term complications of scar contracture and web creep. To recreate the web space, Mondolfi[22] used interdigitating triangular skin flaps and a split thickness skin graft. Weisfeld and Kaplan[23] described a procedure using both dorsal and plantar skin flaps without the use of skin grafts. However, this procedure is not recommended because of the increased chance of vascular compromise.[24] Hikosaka and co-workers[25] reported an open treatment instead of skin graft for partial syndactyly that does not involving the nail pulp of the foot. Open treatment is a technique in which the raw surface is left open to epithelialize, which takes about 5 weeks for wound healing.

We prefer to use a full-thickness skin graft. After reconstruction of an interdigital web with a dorsal flap, the inner wall defect of the smaller toe is covered using a plantar flap, and the lateral wall of the larger toe is covered with a full thickness skin graft. Forceful approximation of the soft tissue defect using local flap may lead to skin necrosis, rotation deformity, or flexion contracture of the digits. Both functional and cosmetic results of syndactyly surgery is satisfactory.

Complications

Three major complications can be encountered: Vascular insufficiency, tension on the area leading to postoperative defects at the surgical site, and digital contractures formed by scar tissue formation.

BRACHYMETATARSIA

Brachymetatarsia is caused by premature arrest of the epiphysis that is caused by congenital or acquired etiology[26–29] and becomes apparent by approximately 10 years of age. A complete physical examination should be performed because the presence of brachymetatarsia may be a manifestation of underlying genetic syndromes and other skeletal deformities. Brachymetatarsia seems to be more problematic in cultures in which shoes are not worn indoors, because this custom exposes the misshapen foot. Most patients who undergo operative correction are female, possibly owing to such cosmetic concerns. Brachymetatarsia can be symptomatic owing to deformity of the involved toe or transfer metatarsalgia to adjacent rays. The incidence of brachymetatarsia is thought to be about 1 in 2000 to 5000.[30] Any metatarsal can be involved; however, the fourth ray is the most frequently affected,[27,31] and the first ray is the second most common.

Symptoms

Patients most often present with concerns of cosmetic appearance. Common symptoms are discomfort from dorsally subluxed toes, which abut the inner surface

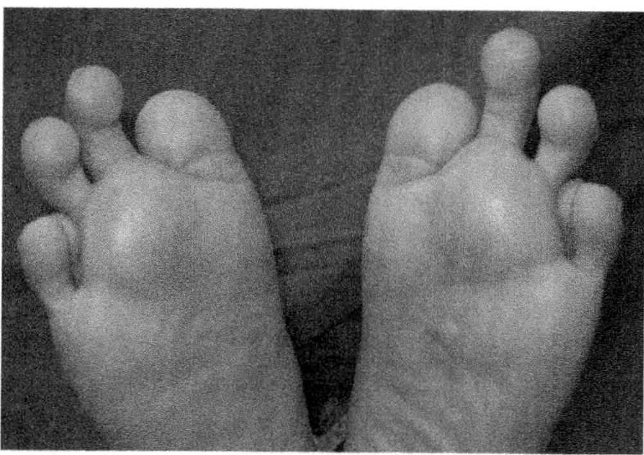

Fig. 10. Callosity under the second and third metatarsal heads in brachymetatarsia of the first and fourth rays.

of the shoe. The skin crease between the third and fourth toes can become symptomatic after prolonged walking. Brachymetatarsia may cause transfer metatarsalgia under the adjacent metatarsal heads[32] (**Fig. 10**). Usually, the symptoms are not so severe as to require surgical correction. Some functional loss may be expected along with improved appearance after surgery. Lengthening of the deficient bone causes frequent complications and a patient should be thoroughly educated about the proper indications for surgical correction.

Treatment

Historically, disarticulation of the symptomatic toe with syndactylization to the adjacent toe is described in the literature. Contemporary reports describe methods for restoring a normal metatarsal parabola by lengthening of the short metatarsal, or a combination procedure with shortening of the longer adjacent metatarsals and lengthening of the short metatarsal[32,33] (**Fig. 11**). Single-stage lengthening by acute intercalary bone graft and gradual distraction lengthening have both been reported.[34–36] When 1-stage lengthening with bone grafting is performed, autogenous iliac bone or allograft can be used as an interposition. When shortening and lengthening are combined, the bone removed during shortening can be used as an autograft for lengthening of the hypoplastic metatarsal.

The main advantages of 1-stage lengthening are that there is no need to apply an external fixator, no possibility of insufficient bone formation, and no need to manipulate the external fixator after surgery. Disadvantages are limitation of lengthening distance,[26,36] and the necessity for bone grafting and immobilization of the metatarsophalangeal joint until union. Allograft instead of autogenous graft might be used without donor site morbidity.[37] The main limitations of 1-stage lengthening are soft tissue tightness, vascular embarrassment, and potential deformity of the toe. Although both 1-stage lengthening and gradual lengthening achieved similar length gains in some reports, the lengthening achieved with 1 stage is smaller than that with gradual lengthening in our experience. Kim and colleagues[26] reported that it is very difficult to lengthen more than 15 mm in a single stage even in younger patients. Ischemia is another concern in 1-stage lengthening. When ischemia persists after waiting more than 15 minutes, removal of longitudinal Kirschner wire after transversely fixing with adjacent metatarsals helps recovery from ischemia (**Fig. 12**). The more frequent problem is the maceration of the plantar aspect of metatarsophalangeal joint (**Fig. 13**). Because of the

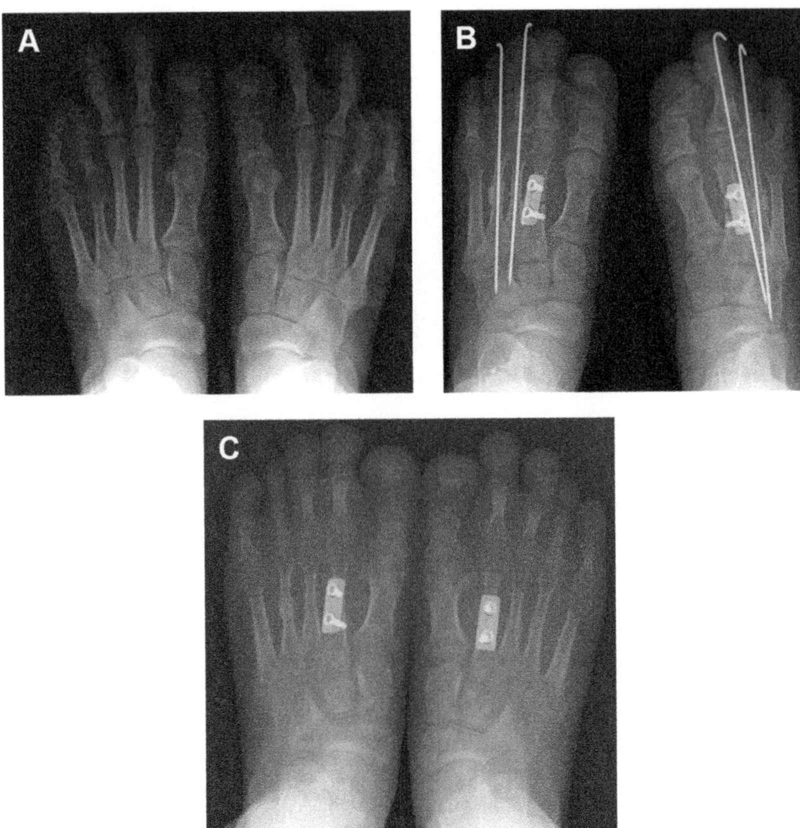

Fig. 11. Improved parabola of the metatarsal heads after combined shortening of the longer metatarsals and lengthening of the shorter metatarsals. Anteroposterior radiograph of the foot: Preoperative (*A*), postoperative (*B*), and at 1-year follow-up (*C*).

plantar slope of the metatarsal, the fourth toe is immobilized in a plantarflexed position, which causes maceration between the skins in the area of skin fold.

The advantages of gradual lengthening are improved lengthening compared with single-stage grafting, immediate weight bearing, and motion of the metatarsophalangeal joint. Distraction osteogenesis in small bones in the feet has been reported to be successful following Illizarov principles.[27,31,36,38–42] Disadvantages are regular manipulation of the external fixator, the possibility of insufficient bone formation, and pin tract infection. To prevent insufficient bone formation, careful osteotomy with minimal soft tissue and vascular damage and strong external fixation is mandatory. Corticotomy in distraction osteogenesis should be performed by minimal traumatic technique to avoid thermal bone damage and to protect the intramedullary vasculature. Osteotomy performed by microsaw has been described as effective, but we have experienced several failures in osteogenesis with this technique and prefer osteotomy by predrilling multiple holes followed by completion with an osteotome.[36] Previous reports[31] indicated that a major risk factor for stiffness of the metatarsophalangeal joint is a large percentage of lengthening, greater than 40%. In our series, the average percentage of lengthening that would result in normal length was a 30% increase.

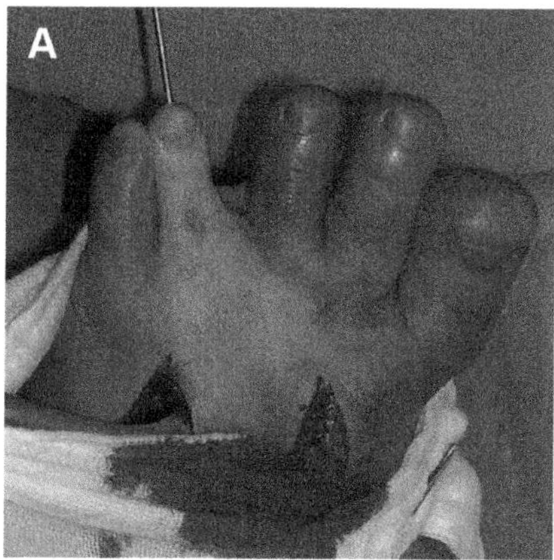

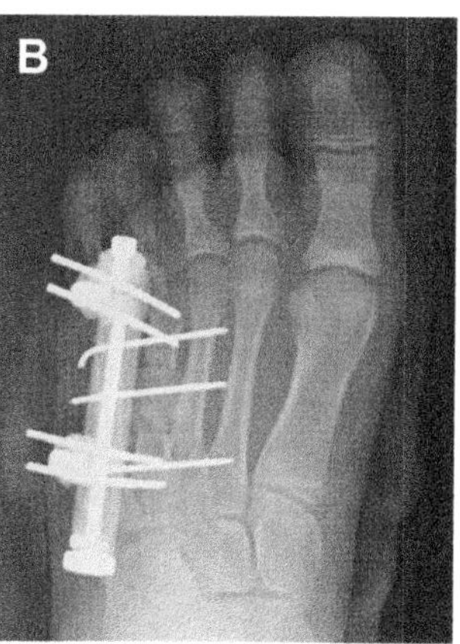

Fig. 12. *A*, Ischemic change of the fourth toe after distraction and immobilization using longitudinal K-wire. *B*, Removal of K-wire and stabilization with external fixator and transverse K-wires.

Hence, there would be little need to lengthen more than 30% of preoperative length, thereby possibly avoiding toe contracture. However, we counsel patients to accept a small amount of shortened appearance to avoid stiffness and toe deformity (**Fig. 14**).

Authors' technique of acute intercalary bone grafting

A dorsal, longitudinal skin incision was made over the fourth metatarsal. After subperiosteal dissection, transverse osteotomy was made with a microsaw at the

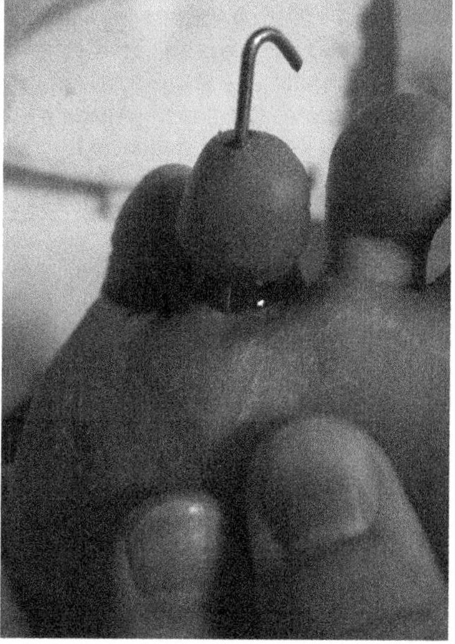

Fig. 13. Exposed K-wire from maceration of skin at the flexion crease of the fourth toe.

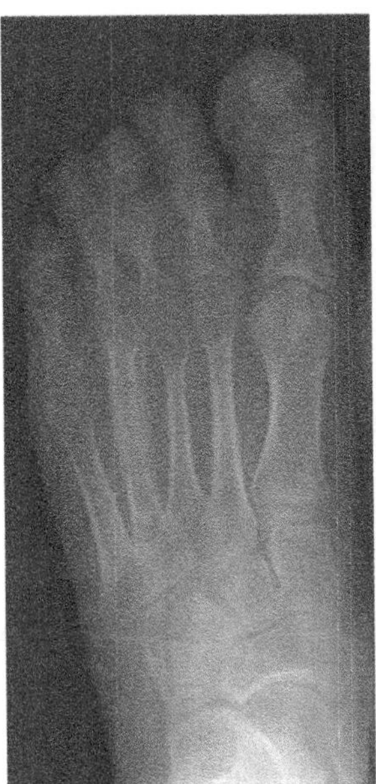

Fig. 14. Anteroposterior radiograph of the foot showing that the head of the fourth metatarsal is more distal to the third metatarsal.

midshaft level. A 0.062-inch Kirschner wire is then driven through the metatarsal head via the osteotomy site of the distal fragment and then antegrade out the tip of the phalanx. The wire is withdrawn until its tip is located distal to the osteotomy site. A lamina spreader is inserted in the osteotomy site and distracted, allowing the opposing surfaces to stretch out the soft tissues for 20 to 30 minutes. An autologous or allograft tricortical iliac bone graft is measured to fill the distracted gap and then the Kirschner wire advanced from the distal fragment across the graft into the proximal metatarsal (**Fig. 15**). A short-leg splint is applied postoperatively and weight bearing on the heel is permitted. To prevent maceration of soft tissue at the flexion crease of the base of the toe, the patient is educated that gauze must be placed deeply in the flexion crease.

Authors' technique of external fixator application and distraction osteotomy of the fourth metatarsal shaft

A dorsal, longitudinal incision is made over the distal half of the metatarsal to expose the neck to midshaft. The periosteum is reflected at the midshaft and the first mini-half-pin inserted at the head neck junction after predrilling with an 0.057-inch Kirschner wire. After a guide was placed with the first mini-half-pin in the most distal hole, the other pins were inserted. A monoplane external fixator (Seoul Meditech, Seoul, Korea) was applied and the osteotomy was created between the second and third mini-half-pins. The authors prefer an osteotomy using a small osteotome after multiple drill holes were made at the site.

All patients are allowed to walk with tolerable weightbearing from the day after surgery. The patients are assessed at 2 weeks for wound examination and education on the distraction method. Distraction commences at the rate of 0.7 mm/d, which is 1 complete turn in the external fixator daily divided into 4 one-quarter turns every 6 hours. Satisfactory results have been reported by distracting 2 to 3 times daily.[42]

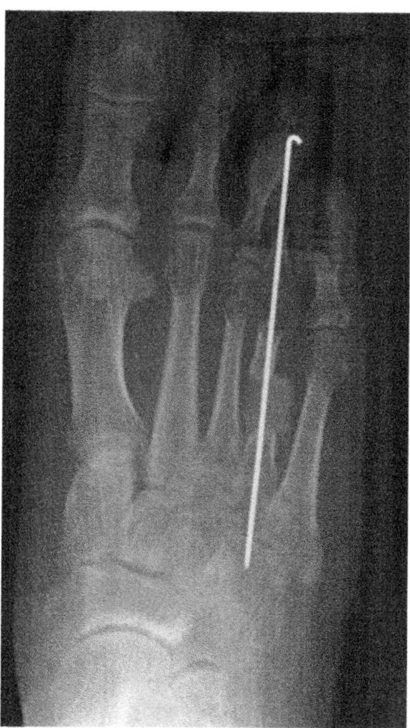

Fig. 15. Anteroposterior radiograph of the foot showing that intercalary graft bone stabilized with a longitudinal K-wire.

Patients are examined again at 10 to 14 days to assess the distraction, and at 3- to 4-week intervals afterward that for radiographic examination. Gauze is tightly wrapped around the mini half pin to prevent motion between the skin and pin (**Fig. 16**). Pain from stretching of the soft tissues appears in almost all patients during lengthening, and the distraction rate can be slowed or temporarily discontinued for several days when there was severe pain.

The fixator is removed in the outpatient clinic after radiographs confirm callus maturation. After external fixator removal, full weightbearing is allowed, but running is not allowed for 4 weeks.

Operative technique for combined shortening and lengthening

The majority of feet are corrected by acute shortening of the second and third metatarsals and lengthening of the fourth. A longitudinal incision is made on the third metatarsal **Fig. 17**. The proximal half of the second metatarsal is exposed through this incision and a transverse osteotomy performed with a microsaw at about 1.5 cm distal to the second metatarsocuneiform joint; the osteotomy cut is made only halfway through the metatarsal. A second osteotomy is performed at a predetermined distance distally, usually 7 to 10 mm distal to the proximal cut, again halfway through the thickness of the metatarsal. Then a hole for 2.7-mm cortical screw was drilled and tapped distal to the distal cut to avoid the difficulty of drilling a hole through the unstable distal fragment after the osteotomy is completed. Then, the osteotomies are completed and a segment of cortical bone removed. Dorsal plating is performed with a 2-hole, one-third semitubular plate or 4-hole narrow plate.

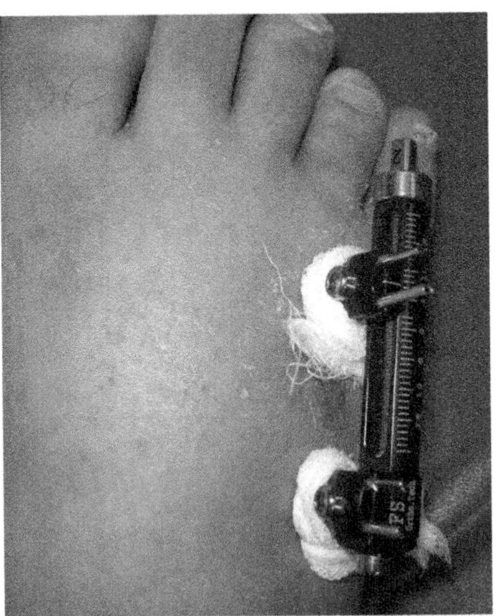

Fig. 16. Gauze tightly wrapped around the pins to prevent motion between skin and pin.

The third metatarsal is exposed and shortened in the same manner; the amount of the shortening is typically 1 or 2 mm shorter than that of the second metatarsal. The third metatarsal can be fixed similarly with plate fixation or alternatively with a longitudinally placed, 0.062-inch K-wire through the phalanges.

The fourth metatarsal is osteotomized through the midshaft and an 0.062-inch K-wire is inserted through the distal fragment to the distal phalanx and withdrawn

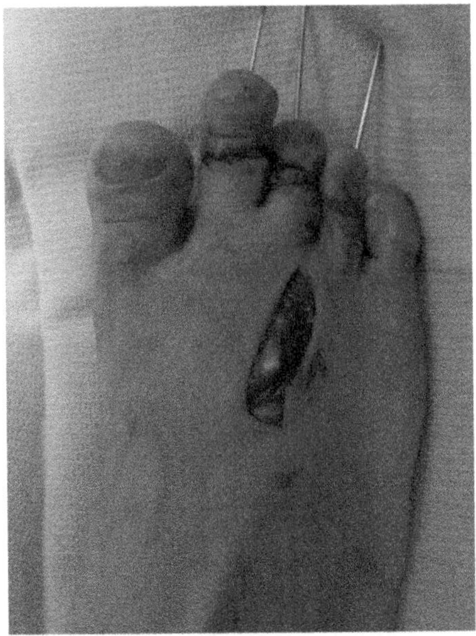

Fig. 17. One incision for combined shortening and lengthening of the second, third, and fourth metatarsals.

distally out until the proximal end of the K-wire is distal to the osteotomy site. Then the osteotomy site is distracted as much as possible by a lamina spreader. The K-wire in the distal fragment is advanced retrograde to the proximal fragment and the cuboid through the interposed bone, which is derived from the second and third metatarsals.

Immediately after surgery, heel weightbearing is allowed and active and passive movement of the second metatarsophalangeal joint encouraged. The K-wire fixing the third metatarsal was removed at the seventh week after the surgery. The K-wire fixing the fourth metatarsal was left in place until some evidence of radiologic evidence of union appeared.

Complications

Stiffness of the MTP joint causes severe functional disability owing to pain and limitation of dorsiflexion, which is essential for normal walking. Stiffness of the first MTP causes more severe functional disability than stiffness of the lesser MTP joints. Stiffness and soft-tissue contracture can occur after excessive lengthening, either acutely or gradually. The authors recommend not lengthening more than a normal parabola, which is the same length of the first and second metatarsal on the

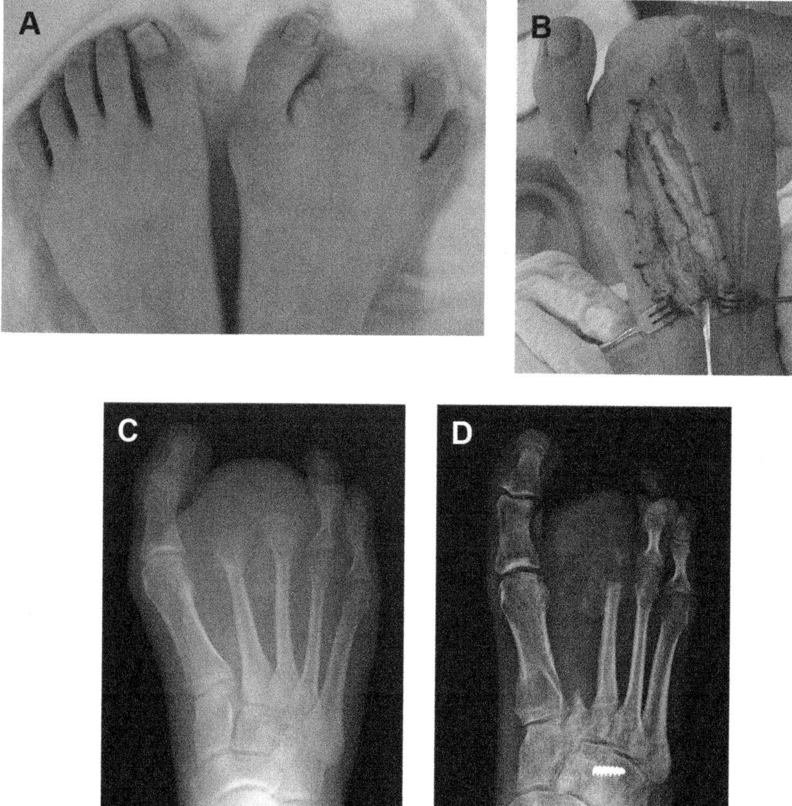

Fig. 18. Macrodactyly. *A*, Right foot macrodactyly in a 20-year-old woman who underwent amputation at age 10. *B*, Intraoperative photograph showing second ray wedge resection. *C*, Preoperative x-ray. *D*, Postoperative x-ray shows a narrowed foot.

dorsoplantar radiograph. We recommend lengthening the fourth metatarsal to a position slightly shorter than the third metatarsal to avoid this complication.

Soft-tissue release for stiffness has been reported, but the results are not well-defined. Our experience with subsequent soft-tissue release is not satisfactory; therefore, we recommend shortening of a lengthened metatarsal if stiffness is severe and persistent.

Angulation at the lengthened segment must be avoided intraoperatively to prevent pressure-related problems. Plantar angulation causes pain at the plantar aspect of the metatarsal head, whereas dorsal malunion leads to transfer metatarsalgia. A shortening osteotomy with removal of a small wedge of bone can correct angular deformities.

MACRODACTYLY

Macrodactyly is a rare congenital anomaly characterized by enlargement of both the soft-tissue and the osseous elements of the toe. The etiology of macrodactyly is obscure and hereditary factors do not seem to be involved.[43] Macrodactyly of the foot differs from macrodactyly of the hand in that there is lower incidence and less involvement of the neural tissue.[44,45] Macrodactyly involved the second and third toes most frequently, with the metatarsal also involved in more than half of the patients.[46]

The timing of operative intervention depends on the severity of the macrodactyly. If it is mild, the patient may be asymptomatic and not regard it as a problem until shoe wear becomes difficult or the toe becomes cosmetically unappealing. In more severe cases, earlier surgery is recommended before full growth of the digit. Delayed surgery does not offer any advantage, and reduction of the width of the foot by ray resection may become more difficult in an adult.[47]

The goal of treatment for macrodactyly of the foot is a painless, cosmetically acceptable foot that can accommodate regular shoes.[46,49] Soft-tissue debulking alone seldom achieves sufficient reduction in the size of the foot,[46–48] and it should be considered a supplemental procedure after bony correction.[46,50] It may also be indicated in skeletally mature patients with mild macrodactyly.

Barsky[43] described 2 types of macrodactyly, one a static type in which an enlargement is present at birth and grows proportionately to the other digits. The other is progressive type in which an enlargement begins in early childhood and grows at a faster rate than the normal digits. He proposed shortening of phalanges by arthrodesis for the treatment of the static type and amputation for the treatment of the progressive type. Ray resection results in a more pleasing cosmetic appearance than does toe amputation at the metatarsophalangeal level.[46,49] When performing a ray resection, additional wedge resection of the cuneiform is good surgical option to reduce the length and the circumference of the foot (**Fig. 18**). Uemura and associates[51] reported a case of second toe macrodactyly that was treated by application of a vascularized nail graft as an island pedicle flap and reconstruct the nail by a 1-stage operation. Because this procedure is usually done in younger patients, parents should be made aware that, as the child matures, the procedure may have to be repeated or multiple operative interventions may be required.

SUMMARY

The treatment of congenital abnormalities of the lesser toes should be individualized to the pathology present. Goals of treatment include pain relief, proper alignment of the toes, and comfort with wearing shoes. Meticulous surgical technique can minimize complications and optimize clinical outcomes for these patients.

REFERENCES

1. Watanabe H, Fujita S, Oka I. Polydactyly of the foot: an analysis of 265 cases and a morphological classification. Plast Reconstr Surg 1992;89:856–77.

2. Nogami H. Polydactyly and polysyndactyly of the fifth toe. Clin Orthop Relat Res 1986;204:261–5.
3. Coppolelli BG, Ready JE, Awbrey BJ, et al. Polydactyly of the foot in adults: literature review and unusual case presentation with diagnostic and treatment recommendations. J Foot Surg 1991;30:12–8.
4. Uda H, Sugawara Y, Niu A, et al. Treatment of lateral ray polydactyly of the foot: focusing on the selection of the toe to be excised. Plast Reconstr Surg 2002;109:1581–91.
5. Morley SE, Smith PJ. Polydactyly of the feet in children: suggestions for surgical management. Br J Plast Surg 2001;54:34–8.
6. Phelps DA, Grogan DP. Polydactyly of the foot. J Pediatr Orthop 1985;5:446–51.
7. Allen BL Jr. Plantar-advancement skin flap for central ray resections in the foot: description of a technique. J Pediatr Orthop 1997;17:785–9.
8. Shaheed N, Nealy JA, Bituin BV. A rare occurrence of polydactyly. J Am Podiatr Med Assoc 2000;90:425–9.
9. Kazuhiro Masada, Y Tsuyuguchi, H Kawabata, et al. Treatment of preaxial polydactyly of the foot. Plast Reconstr Surg 1987;79:251–8.
10. Temtamy S, McKusick VA. Synopsis of hand malformations with particular emphasis on genetic factors. Birth Defects 1969;5:125–84.
11. Venn-Watson E. Problems in polydactyly of the foot. Orthop Clin North Am 1976;7: 909–27.
12. Lee HS, Park SS, Youm YS, et al. Classification of postaxial polydactyly of the foot. Foot Ankle Int 2006; 27:356–62.
13. Nakamura K, Nanjyo B, Yoshii M. Postaxial polydactylies of the lower limb. Jpn J Plast Reconstr Surg 1989;32:233.
14. Coleman WB, Kissel CG, Sterling HD Jr. Syndactylism and its surgical repair. J Am Podiatry Assoc. 1981;71:545–50.
15. Hancock PA, Flory RJ. Syndactyly. A review of the literature. J Am Podiatry Assoc 1974;64:25–34.
16. Kettelkamp DB, Flatt AE. An evaluation of syndactylia repair. Surg Gynecol Obstet 1961;113:471–8.
17. Mempel M, Abeck D, Lange I, et al. The wide spectrum of clinical expression in Adams-Oliver syndrome: a report of two cases. Br J Dermatol 1999;140:1157–60.
18. Vogels A, Fryns JP. Pfeiffer syndrome. Orphanet J Rare Dis 2006;1:19.
19. Baris H, Tan WH, Kimonis VE. Hypothelia, syndactyly, and ear malformation: a variant of the scalp-ear-nipple syndrome? Case report and review of the literature. Am J Med Genet A 2005;134A:220–2.
20. Patrizi A, Neri I, Fiorentini C, Marzaduri S. Nevus comedonicus syndrome: a new pediatric case. Pediatr Dermatol 1998;15:304–6.
21. Shimizu H, Sato M, Ban M, et al. Immunohistochemical, ultrastructural, and molecular features of Kindler syndrome distinguish it from dystrophic epidermolysis bullosa. Arch Dermatol 1997;133:1111–7.
22. Mondolfi PE. Syndactyly of the toes. Plast Reconstr Surg 1983;71:212–8.
23. Weisfeld M, Kaplan EG. Surgical treatment of congenital zygodactylism and brachymetapody: a case history. J Foot Surg 1977;16:24–34.
24. Juris RS, Kanat IO. Desyndactyly: a literature review. J Foot Surg 1990;29:463–70.
25. Hikosaka M, Ogata H, Nakajima T, et al. Advantages of open treatment for syndactyly of the foot: defining its indications. Scand J Plast Reconstr Surg Hand Surg 2009;28:1–5.
26. Kim HT, Lee SH, Yoo CI, et al. The management of brachymetatarsia. J Bone Joint Surg Br 2003;85:683–90.

27. Shim JS, Park SJ. Treatment of brachymetatarsia by distraction osteogenesis. J Pediatr Orthop 2006;26:250–4.
28. Sinclair GG, Shoemaker SK, Seibert SR. Iatrogenic brachymetatarsia. J Foot Surg 1991;30:580.
29. Saxby T, Nunley JN. Metatarsal lengthening by distraction osteogenesis: a report of two cases. Foot Ankle 1992;13:536–9.
30. Urano Y, Kobayachi A. Bone-lengthening for shortness of the fourth toe. J Bone Joint Surg Am 1978;60:91–3.
31. Masada K, Fujita S, Fuji T, et al. Complications following metatarsal lengthening by callus distraction for brachymetatarsia. J Pediatr Orthop 1999;19:394–7.
32. Lee WC, Suh JS, Moon JS, et al. Treatment of brachymetatarsia of the first and fourth ray in adults. Foot Ankle Int 2009;30:981–5.
33. Kim JS, Baek GH, Chung MS, et al. Multiple congenital brachymetatarsia. A one-stage combined shortening and lengthening procedure without iliac bone graft. J Bone Joint Surg Br 2004;86:1013–5.
34. Choi IH, Chung MS, Baek GH, et al. Metatarsal lengthening in congenital brachymetatarsia: one-stage lengthening versus lengthening by callotasis. J Pediatr Orthop 1999;19:660–4.
35. Baek GH, Chung MS. The treatment of congenital brachymetatarsia by one-stage lengthening. J Bone Joint Surg Br 1998;80:1040–4.
36. Lee WC, Yoo JH, Moon JS. Lengthening of fourth brachymetatarsia by three different surgical techniques. J Bone Joint Surg Br 2009;91:1472–7.
37. Giannini S, Faldini C, Pagkrati S, et al. One-stage metatarsal lengthening by allograft interposition: a novel approach for congenital brachymetatarsia. Clin Orthop Relat Res 2010;468:1933–42.
38. Levine SE, Davidson RS, Dormans JP, et al. Distraction osteogenesis for congenitally short lesser metatarsals. Foot Ankle Int 1995;16:196–200.
39. Hurst JM, Nunley JA 2nd. Distraction osteogenesis for the shortened metatarsal after hallux valgus surgery. Foot Ankle Int 2007;28:194–8.
40. Wada A, Bensahel H, Takamura K, et al. Metatarsal lengthening by callus distraction for brachymetatarsia. J Pediatr Orthop B 2004;13:206–10.
41. Song HR, Oh CW, Kyung HS, et al. Fourth brachymetatarsia treated with distraction osteogenesis. Foot Ankle Int 2003;24:706–11.
42. Lee KB, Park HW, Chung JY, et al. Comparison of the outcomes of distraction osteogenesis for first and fourth brachymetatarsia. J Bone Joint Surg Am 2010;92:2709–18.
43. Barsky AJ. Macrodactyly. J Bone Joint Surg Am 1967;49:1255–66.
44. Kalen V, Burwell DS, Omer GE. Macrodactyly of the hands and feet. J Pediatr Orthop 1988;8:311–5.
45. Tsuge K. Treatment of macrodactyly. Plast Reconstr Surg 1967;39:590–9.
46. Chang CH, Kumar SJ, Riddle EC, et al. Macrodactyly of the foot. J Bone Joint Surg Am 2002;84:1189–94.
47. Rechnagel K. Megalodactylism. Report of 7 cases. Acta Orthop Scand 1967;38:57–66.
48. Dedrick D, Kling TF Jr. Ray resection in the treatment of macrodactyly of the foot in children. Orthop Trans 1985;9:145.
49. Ahn JH, Choy WS, Kim HY, et al. Treatment of macrodactyly in the adult foot: a case report. Foot Ankle Int 2008;29:1253–7.
50. Kotwal PP, Farooque M. Macrodactyly. J Bone Joint Surg Br 1998;80:651–3.
51. Uemura T, Kazuki K, Okada M, et al. A case of toe macrodactyly treated by application of a vascularised nail graft. Br J Plast Surg 2005;58:1020–4.

Bunionette Deformity: Etiology, Nonsurgical Management, and Lateral Exostectomy

Todd Bertrand, MD[a], Selene G. Parekh, MD, MBA[b,c,*]

KEYWORDS

- Bunionette • Coughlin series
- Fourth–fifth intermetatarsal angle • Lateral exostectomy

Bunionette is a term used to characterize a lateral prominence of the fifth metatarsal head. Also known as a "tailor's bunion," due to the cross-legged position of a tailor, the bunionette deformity usually consists of both an abnormal fifth metatarsal as well as overlying soft tissues.[1] Bunionettes can occur in many individuals and are often noted as incidental findings. Very rarely do these become significant enough to warrant treatment.

Increased pressure over the lateral condyle of the fifth metatarsal head can lead to chronic irritation of the overlying bursa.[2] Friction between an underlying bony abnormality and constricting footwear may lead to the development of a keratosis over the lateral or plantar lateral aspect of the fifth metatarsal head.[2] Varus deviation of the fifth toe at the metatarsophalangeal joint leads to focal pressure over the lateral eminence, also contributing to pain and callus formation.

ETIOLOGY

In contrast to prior descriptions, the bunionette deformity is not analogous to the medial eminence of the first metatarsal head in a hallux valgus deformity.[2] The fifth metatarsal normally deviates from the fourth by approximately 5°. In addition, the head of the fifth metatarsal is often broader than the shaft. This can lead to a lateral prominence that causes pain with tight footwear. The etiology of bunionette deformities can be divided into two broad categories: *anatomic* and *biomechanical*.[3]

The authors have nothing to disclose for this project and paper.
[a] Department of Orthopaedic Surgery, Duke University School of Medicine, Durham, NC 27710, USA
[b] Department of Orthopaedic Surgery, North Carolina Orthopaedic Clinic, 3609 Southwest Durham Drive Durham, NC 27707, USA
[c] Fuqua School of Business, Duke University, 100 Fuqua Drive Durham, NC 27708, USA
* Corresponding author. Department of Orthopaedic Surgery, North Carolina Orthopaedic Clinic, 3609 Southwest Durham Drive Durham, NC 27707.
E-mail address: selene.parekh@gmail.com

Foot Ankle Clin N Am 16 (2011) 679–688
doi:10.1016/j.fcl.2011.08.003
foot.theclinics.com

Anatomic causes could include the following:

- Tight footwear causing pressure over the lateral fifth metatarsal
- Abnormal foot position (lateral aspect of the foot resting on the ground)
- Prominent lateral fifth metatarsal head
- Hypertrophy of soft tissues overlying lateral aspect of the fifth metatarsal head
- "Dumbbell"-shaped fifth metatarsal
- Supernumerary ossicles attached to the lateral fourth metatarsal, pushing the fifth metatarsal laterally
- Increased fourth–fifth intermetatarsal angle (splaying)
- Incomplete insertion or development of the transverse metatarsal ligament.

Biomechanical causes could include the following:

- Lateral bending/deviation of the fifth metatarsal
- Congenital plantar or dorsiflexed fifth ray deformities
- Excessive pronation due to hypermobility of the fifth metatarsal
- Subluxatory pronation of the fifth metatarsal (associated with pronation of subtalar and midtarsal joints)
- Pes planus (hindfoot eversion leads to a more laterally pronounced fifth metatarsal).

CLINICAL PRESENTATION

A bunionette deformity is commonly seen in adolescents and adults, with a female/male ratio reported to be anywhere between 1:1 and 10:1.[3] Regardless of the underlying anatomy, the common symptom that all patients with a bunionette deformity note is increased pressure over the fifth metatarsal head due to constricting footwear.[2] The increased occurrence of bunionette deformity in the female population is most likely secondary to a predilection for fashionable footwear (**Fig. 1**). Swelling of the soft tissues overlying the lateral aspect of the fifth metatarsal head can lead to pain.

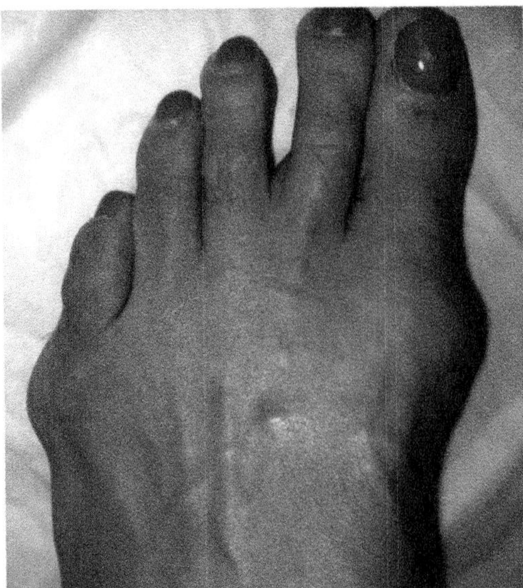

Fig. 1. A 60-year-old woman with lateral-sided foot pain associated with shoe wear (Adapted from Cohen BE, Nicholson CW. Bunionette deformity. J Am Acad Orthop Surg 2007;15:300–7. © 2007 American Academy of Orthopaedic Surgeons. Reprinted with permission.)

Three distinct areas of pain have been described in relation to the head of fifth metatarsal: laterally, dorsolaterally, and plantarly. The location of the callosity is important, as this will guide treatment. Patients with a bunionette deformity will often present with erythema and edema over a deformity on the lateral aspect of the foot. In immunocompromised patients, rarely ulceration can occur that can lead to superinfection. Over time, as continuous pressure is applied over the lateral aspect of the fifth metatarsal, a secondary hyperkeratotic lesion can develop over the lateral or plantar aspects of the fifth toe. This hyperkeratosis can occasionally cause the fifth toe to deviate medially at the metatarsophalangeal joint while the metatarsal deviates laterally.

IMAGING

Radiographically, standard weight-bearing views of the foot are obtained, including dorsoplantar, lateral, and oblique. For the dorsoplantar view, the source of the x-ray should be 12 in (30 cm) above the foot and tilted 15°. Lateral radiographs should be made with the cassette along the medial aspect of the foot. The x-ray source should be perpendicular to the cassette and approximately 48 in (120 cm) away. Oblique radiographs are helpful in evaluation the fifth metatarsal head, lateral tubercle, metatarsal deviation, and lateral soft tissue prominence (**Fig. 2**).

The fourth–fifth intermetatarsal (4–5 IM) angle calculates the divergence of the fourth and fifth metatarsals. It is formed by the intersection of two lines that bisect the

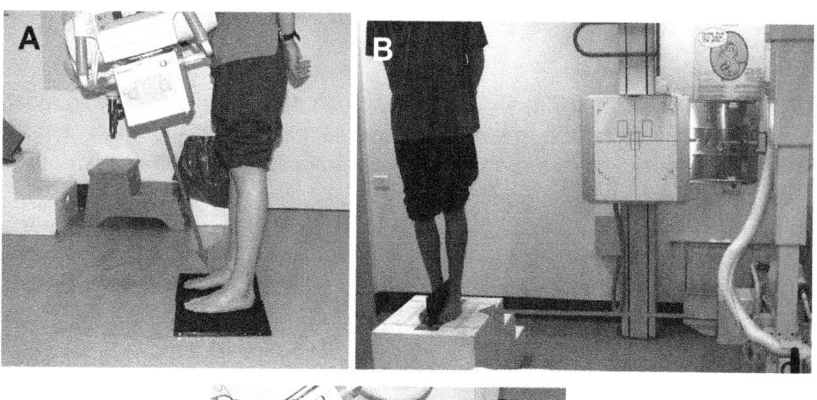

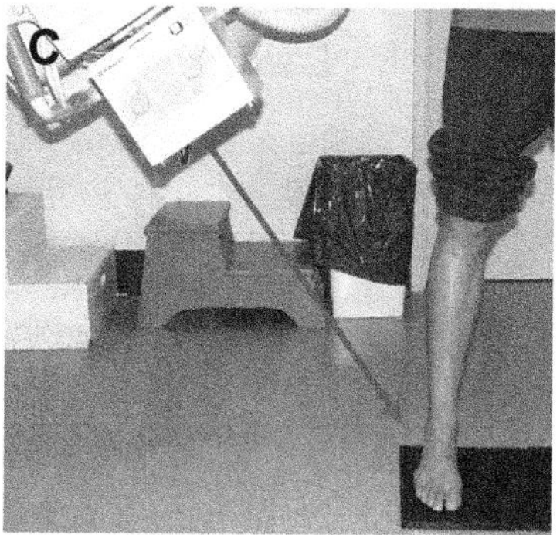

Fig. 2. Technique for weight-bearing images of the foot: AP (*A*), lateral (*B*), oblique (*C*).

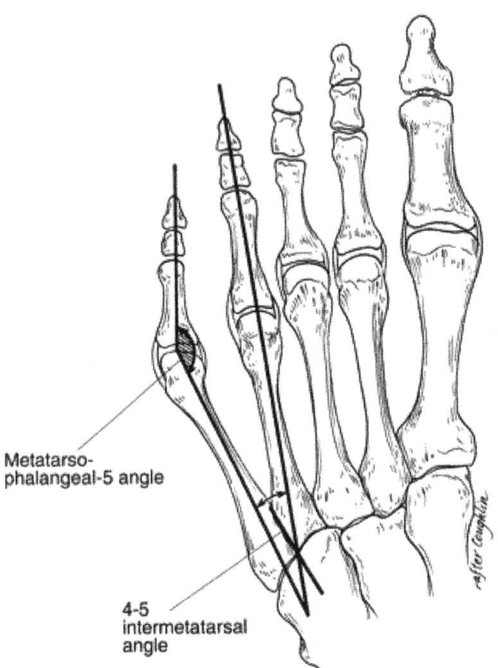

Fig. 3. Technique for measuring the 4–5 IM angle and the fifth metatarsophalangeal angle. (Adapted from Cohen BE, Nicholson CW. Bunionette deformity. J Am Acad Orthop Surg 2007; 15:300–7. © 2007 American Academy of Orthopaedic Surgeons. Reprinted with permission.)

fourth and fifth metatarsals (**Fig. 3**). Another method of measuring has been reported that involves a line along the medial and proximal portions of the shaft of the fifth metatarsal. Divergence of the fourth and fifth metatarsals may result in a symptomatic fifth metatarsal head lesion.

The normal 4–5 IM angle is 6.5° (range, 3–11°) in patients without a bunionette and 9.6° in feet with a symptomatic bunionette.[4] However, Coughlin noted the preoperative 4–5 IM angle in symptomatic patients to be 10.6°.[5] In patients with pes planus, the 4–5 IM angle may be increased by up to 3°.[4] In general, a 4–5 IM angle greater than 8° is felt to be abnormal.[2] However, in asymptomatic individuals, surgical intervention may not be required.

The fifth metatarsophalangeal angle indicates the magnitude of medial deviation of the fifth toe in relation to the axis of the fifth metatarsal[2] (**Fig. 3**). In 90% of normal feet, this angle is 14° or less (range, 1–21°).[6] The mean fifth metatarsophalangeal angle in patients with symptomatic bunionette is 16° (range, 5 to 30°).[5]

Lateral bowing, or deviation, of the fifth toe is often associated with a bunionette deformity. The degree of lateral bowing, which often occurs at the distal third of the fifth metatarsal shaft, is termed the lateral deviation angle. This is measured on the dorsoplantar radiograph by an angle formed from a line bisecting the midpoint of the articular surface of the metatarsal head and neck to the metatarsal base and a line drawn parallel to the medial cortex of the proximal metatarsal (**Fig. 4**). The average lateral deviation angle is 2.6° (range, 0–7°) in normal feet and 8° (range, 4–14°) in patients with a bunionette deformity.[4]

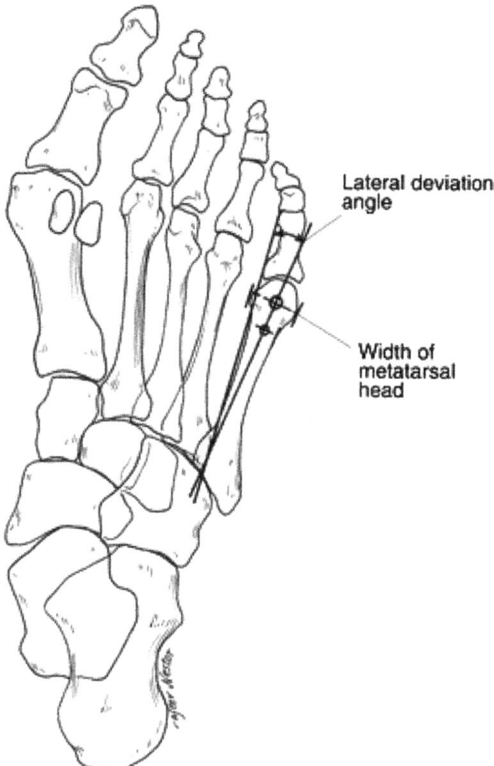

Fig. 4. Technique for measuring the lateral deviation angle. (Adapted from Cohen BE, Nicholson CW. Bunionette deformity. J Am Acad Orthop Surg 2007;15:300–7. © 2007 American Academy of Orthopaedic Surgeons. Reprinted with permission.)

The normal width of the fifth metatarsal head is less than 13 mm.[7] Prominence of the fifth metatarsal head may also be due to pronation of the foot with lateral rotation of the lateral tubercle.[4,8]

CLASSIFICATION

Four types of bunionette deformity have been described; however, the three types described by Coughlin are traditionally used.[4,5] The classification is based on weight-bearing dorsoplantar radiographs (**Fig. 5**):

Type I is an enlargement of the lateral surface of the fifth metatarsal. This could be secondary to an exostosis; a prominent lateral condyle; or a round, or dumbbell-shaped, metatarsal head. It has been observed that with excessive pronation of the foot, the lateral plantar tubercle of the fifth metatarsal head rotates laterally to create the radiographic impression of an enlarged fifth metatarsal head.[2,4]

Type II is secondary to abnormal lateral bowing of the distal fifth metatarsal with a normal 4–5 IM angle. There is usually not associated hypertrophy of the fifth metatarsal head.

Type III, the most common in Coughlin's series, is characterized by an increased 4–5 IM angle with divergence of the fourth and fifth metatarsals.

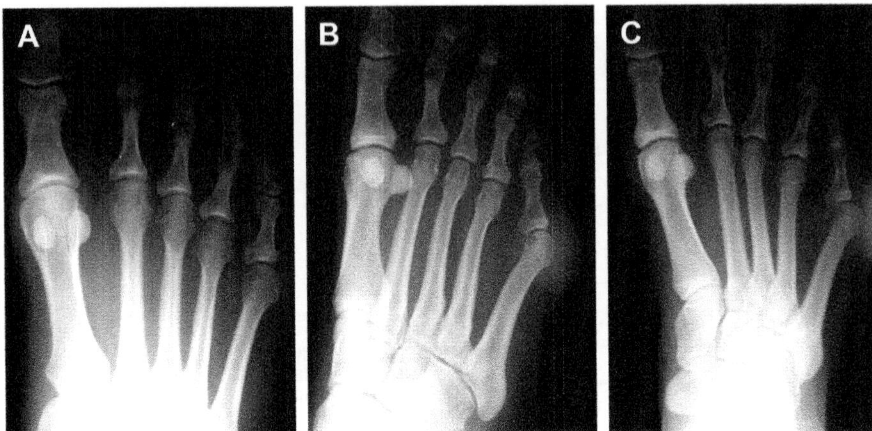

Fig. 5. Weight-bearing dorsoplantar radiographs demonstrating bunionette classification. (*A*) Type I, with lateral prominence of the fifth metatarsal head. (*B*) Type II, with lateral bowing of the fifith metatarsal. (*C*) Type III, with widening of the 4–5 IM angle. (Adapted from Cohen BE, Nicholson CW. Bunionette deformity. J Am Acad Orthop Surg 2007;15:300–7. © 2007 American Academy of Orthopaedic Surgeons. Reprinted with permission.)

Type IV, not described by Coughlin, is not common and consists of a combination of deformities including two or more of the types listed above. This is most commonly seen in the feet of patients with rheumatoid arthritis.

In Coughlin's series of symptomatic bunionette deformities corrected by metatarsal diaphyseal osteotomy, a type I deformity was noted in 27% of cases, a type II deformity in 23% of cases, and type III in 50% of cases.[2,5]

CONSERVATIVE (NONSURGICAL) MANAGEMENT

No evidence-based guidelines exist for the conservative management of bunionette deformity; however, there are several agreed upon recommendations. Nonsurgical management should be considered initially for all bunionette deformities. Conservative care is often successful in treating symptomatic bunionette, with reports of only 10% to 23% requiring surgical intervention.[7,9] Constricting footwear is a significant cause of symptoms and places increased pressure on a prominent fifth metatarsal head.

Initial management should include wearing shoes with a wider toe-box, as most patients have pain only with shoe wear. Shoes can also be altered to accommodate the lateral deformity, including cutouts or stretching. Inflamed soft tissues overlying a bunionette deformity may be managed with felt or silicone gel pads. Hyperkeratotic lesions can be periodically pared down and padded to help alleviate pain. If the bunionette is associated with other deformities, including pes planus, orthotic devices may be helpful in reducing pronation. A larger shoe size may be necessary to accommodate these devices. Nonsteroidal oral analgesics and corticosteroid injections have been reportedly used in patients with an acutely inflamed bursa overlying the fifth metatarsal head without adverse side effects.[3]

SURGICAL MANAGEMENT

Operative management is warranted in patients with symptomatic bunionette deformity who have not responded to nonsurgical treatment or in patients with special demands, such as high-performing athletes. Recognition of the specific anatomic variation present is important in the preoperative evaluation, as this may influence the specific surgical procedure chosen.[2] Operative procedures can be divided into exostectomies, resections, and various metatarsal osteotomies. Metatarsal osteotomies can be divided based upon the anatomic location: proximal, diaphyseal, or distal. Other options that have been described but are of limited usefulness are metatarsal head resection, fifth metatarsal ray resection, and isolated soft tissue procedures.

The goals of surgical intervention are to decrease the width of the forefoot as well as the prominence of the bunionette. Correction of the underlying pathology is necessary to prevent a recurrence of the deformity. Likewise, preservation of function of the fifth metatarsophalangeal joint may prevent such complications as recurrence, subluxation, dislocation, or the development of a transfer lesion.[2]

Lateral Exostectomy

A lateral exostectomy may be performed to alleviate an isolated enlargement of the fifth metatarsal head or prominent fifth metatarsal lateral condyle without an increased 4–5 IM angle. Lateral exostectomy is most often indicated for type I deformities with a lateral callosity. Several procedures have been described, including resection of the lateral third of the fifth metatarsal head as well as resection of the entire fifth metatarsal head. The goal of the procedure is to remove the lateral prominence associated with the bunionette and narrow the width of the forefoot. By removing the lateral condyle of the fifth metatarsal head, the 4–5 IM angle is not changed. Further, simple exostectomy is preferable to osteotomy in some situations in which patients are unable to restrict weight bearing on the lateral aspect of their forefoot and whose main preoperative complaint is pain secondary to a prominent lateral condyle.

A simple lateral exostectomy is not effective for bunionettes with associated intractable plantar keratosis under the fifth metatarsal head, as the exostectomy does not address plantar pressure. The presence of pes planus or forefoot pronation is considered a relative contraindication as the pressure will continue due to position of the hindfoot and forefoot. Other disadvantages to simple exostectomy that have been reported include recurrence of deformity, joint instability, and production of an incongruous joint with possible lateral dislocation of the fifth metatarsophalangeal joint.

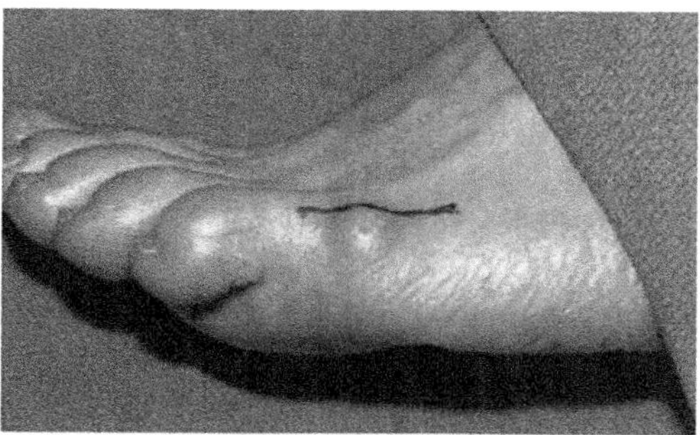

Fig. 6. Dorsolateral skin incision over the lateral condyle of the fifth metatarsal head.

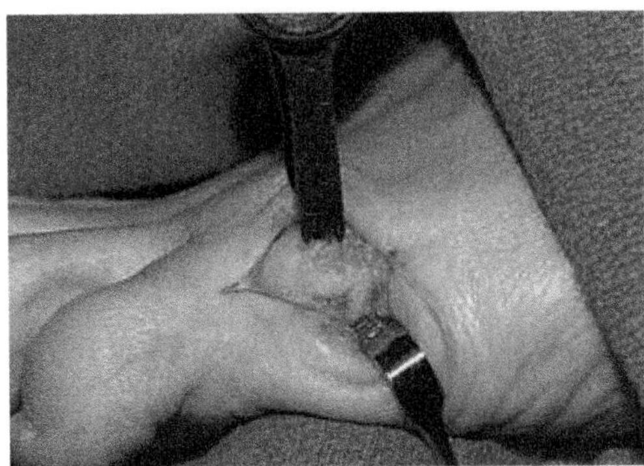

Fig. 7. Capsular incision is made allowing identification of the lateral condylar process of the fifth metatarsal head.

Surgical procedure

A 2- to 3-cm skin incision is made in a longitudinal fashion over the lateral condyle of the fifth metatarsal head, extending from the metatarsophalangeal joint to 1 cm. distal to the fifth metatarsal condyle[2] (**Fig. 6**).

The subcutaneous tissues are gently retracted. The lateral dorsal cutaneous nerve of the fifth toe should be identified and protected. Early identification of this nerve before capsulotomy may help avoid a painful incisional neuroma. The joint capsule of the fifth metatarsophalangeal joint is identified and an inverted "L" capsular incision is made (**Fig. 7**).

The proximal and dorsal limbs of the capsule are detached. The dorsal and proximal limbs are the weakest part of the capsule, therefore leaving the stronger plantar and distal limbs attached.[2] Excessive soft tissue stripping off the fifth metatarsal head should be avoided so as to not affect the blood supply. The lateral condylar process of the fifth metatarsal is then identified. Resection of the lateral condylar process occurs in a plane that parallels the lateral border of the foot, using a microsagittal saw with a thin saw blade (**Fig. 8**).

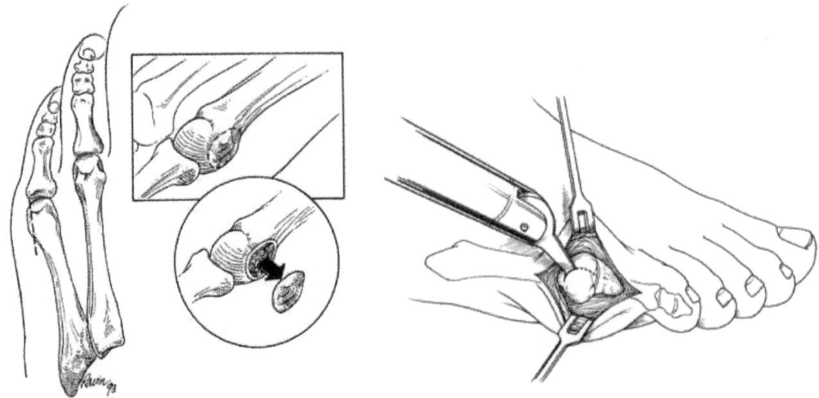

Fig. 8. Resection of lateral condylar process of the fifth metatarsal head parallels the lateral border of the foot.

With traction placed on the fifth toe, the metatarsophalangeal joint is distracted and the medial capsule is released with a scalpel.[2]

The metatarsophalangeal joint capsule is closed by reapproximation to the fifth metatarsal periosteum as well as to the abductor digiti quinti muscle proximally. If improved fixation is warranted, the capsule may be anchored through drill holes in the dorsolateral metaphysis of the fifth metatarsal. A meticulous repair of the joint capsule is necessary to prevent recurrence of the deformity or lateral subluxation of the metatarsophalangeal joint. The skin is closed in routine fashion and a compressive dressing is applied.[2]

Postoperatively, the patient is allowed to ambulate in a postoperative shoe for 3 weeks and then in a sandal for 3 weeks. Skin sutures are removed 2 to 3 weeks after surgery.

Results of lateral exostectomy

In the only long-term evaluation of lateral exostectomy for bunionette deformity, Kitaoko and colleagues performed 21 lateral condylar resections in 16 patients with a symptomatic bunionette. In an average follow-up of 6.4 years, 71% of patients were satisfied with their results. The average forefoot score improved from 40.3 $\pm$ 13.5

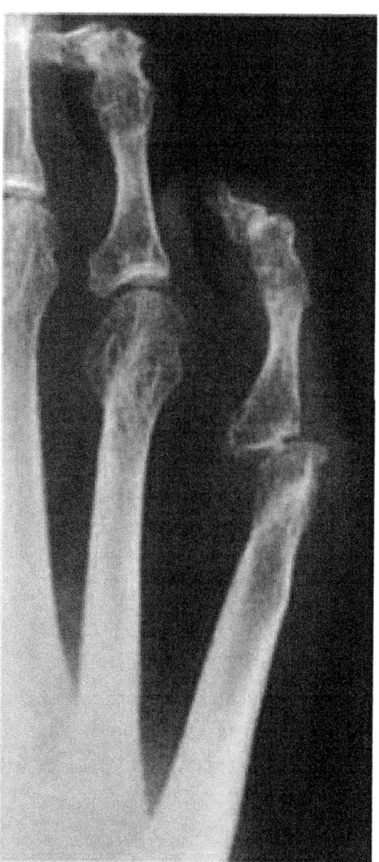

Fig. 9. AP radiograph of a painful recurrent bunionette after lateral condylar resection. Note the medial deviation of the fifth toe.

points to 68.3 ± 11.7 points out of a possible 75 points. Twenty-three percent of patients reported some element of forefoot pain, although half of these considered it mild. The 4–5 IM angle and the fifth metatarsophalangeal angle did not change significantly. In two cases, the metatarsophalangeal joint subluxated postoperatively, as the fifth toe displaced medially. Based upon this, it was recommended that a tight capsular closure be performed with excision of redundant joint capsule. In the presence of an intractable plantar keratosis beneath the fifth metatarsal head, the authors felt a simple condylectomy was contraindicated. The authors concluded that although lateral exostectomy was limited in correcting the deformity present, it was often successful in relieving symptoms.[10]

Complications of lateral exostectomy

Complications following lateral exostectomy for bunionette deformity have been reported in the literature. Some of these include fifth metatarsophalangeal joint subluxation, recurrence of deformity, poor weight bearing with excessive lateral condylar resection, fifth toe hypesthesia, and infection.

Fifth metatarsophalangeal joint subluxation is most often secondary to inadequate capsular repair. If the dorsal and proximal limbs of the capsule are not adequately repaired with removal of any redundant capsular tissue, the fifth toe will tend to deviate medially (**Fig. 9**). This is prevented by a meticulous capsular closure as well as attention to repair of the abductor digiti quinti.[2]

The significant recurrence rate following lateral exostectomy is due to the use of this procedure when a fifth metatarsal osteotomy is indicated. The only indication for a lateral exostectomy is a symptomatic enlarged lateral condyle.[2] When a metatarsal osteotomy is indicated from the preoperative radiographs for correction of the deformity, a lateral exostectomy may produce only temporary results, with the bunionette recurring over time.

REFERENCES

1. Cohen BE, Nicholson CW. Bunionette deformity. J Am Acad Orthop Surg 2007; 15:300–7.
2. Mann RA, Coughlin MJ. Surgery of the foot and ankle. 6th edition. St. Louis (MO): CV Mosby; 1993.
3. Kotti M, Maffulli N. Bunionette. J Bone Joint Surg Am 2001;83:1076–82.
4. Fallat LM, Buckholz J. An analysis of the tailor's bunion by radiographic and anatomical display. J Am Podiatr Assoc 1980;70:597–603.
5. Coughlin MJ. Treatment of bunionette deformity with longitudinal diaphyseal with distal soft tissue repair. Foot Ankle 1991;11:195–203.
6. Steel MW 3rd, Johnson KA, DeWitz MA, Ilstrup DM. Radiographic measurements of the normal adult foot. Foot Ankle 1980;1:151–8.
7. Nestor BJ, Kitaoka HB, Ilstrup DM, et al. Radiologic anatomy of the painful bunionette. Foot Ankle 1990;11:6–11.
8. Gerbert J, Sgarlato TE, Subotnick SI. Preliminary study of a closing wedge osteotomy of the fifth metatarsal for correction of a tailor's bunion deformity. J Am Podiatry Assoc 1972;62:212–8.
9. Diebold PF. Basal osteotomy of the fifth metatarsal for the bunionette. Foot Ankle. 1991;12:74–9.
10. Kitaoko HB, Holiday AD Jr. Lateral condylar resection for bunionette. Clin Orthop Relat Res 1992;May(278):183–92.

Osteotomies for Bunionette Deformity

Lowell Weil Jr, DPM*, Lowell Scott Weil Sr, DPM

KEYWORDS

- Bunionette • Osteotomy • Scarfette
- Surgical decision making • Minimal incision surgery
- Tailors bunion

A tailor's bunion or bunionette deformity is a combination of an osseous and soft-tissue bursitis located on the lateral aspect of the fifth metatarsal head and was first described by Davies[1] as a condition caused by splaying of the fifth metatarsal. The condition is often present with hallux valgus deformity, both of which are noted with a flexible splayfoot (**Fig. 1**).

Chronic shoe pressure over the lateral part of the fifth metatarsal head leads to hypertrophy of the overlying soft tissue; bursal thickening; and less often, localized hyperkeratosis. In the presence of hallux valgus deformity, the width of the forefoot is increased, thereby causing increased pressure on the lateral side of the fifth metatarsal head. The cause of the deformity of the fifth metatarsal head can be from a localized, enlarged bony prominence but most often the true etiology is a rotational movement of the fifth ray at its articulation with the cuboid. The fifth ray excessively pronates, leading to a progressive deformity that is accompanied by the fifth toe seeking an adducto-varus position.[2–4] The condition can also occur as a result of a structural deformity with both plantar flexion and abduction of the fifth ray, producing a plantar keratosis as well as a bunionette deformity. The plantar keratosis condition is most frequently seen in a cavus foot type.[5]

As in hallux valgus deformity, several retrospective studies indicate that the condition is between 3 and 10 times more common in women than in men and has a peak incidence during the fourth and fifth decades of life.[2,6]

Conservative treatments may resolve some of the associated bursitis or fifth metatarsal–phalangeal joint, but will not likely create any long-term benefits.[2]

SURGICAL PLANNING

In 1990, Fallat and Bucholz[7] described a classification system for surgical management of symptomatic tailor's bunion. Type 1 is an enlargement of the lateral aspe5ct of the fifth metatarsal head; type 2, a lateral bowing of the distal aspect of the

The authors have nothing to disclose.
Weil Foot & Ankle Institute, 1455 Golf Road, Des Plaines, IL 60016, USA
* Corresponding author.
E-mail address: lwj@weil4feet.com

Foot Ankle Clin N Am 16 (2011) 689–712
doi:10.1016/j.fcl.2011.08.012
foot.theclinics.com
1083-7515/11/$ – see front matter

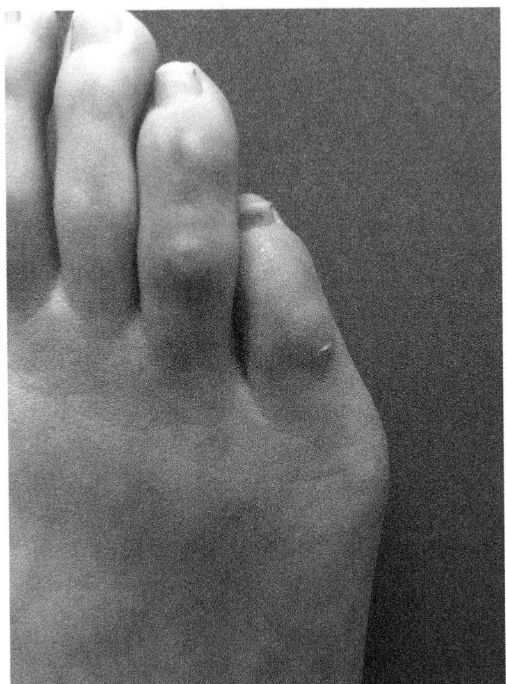

Fig. 1. Classic bunionette deformity.

pronated fifth metatarsal; type 3, an increased fourth–fifth intermetatarsal angle (4–5 IMA); and type 4, a combination of two or more deformities. Coughlin[8] postulated that these criteria should enable the surgeon to better recognize the type of bunionette deformity and assist in the choice of an appropriate surgical technique.

A key radiographic measurement associated with a bunionette deformity is the intermetatarsal angle between the fourth and fifth metatarsals, which normally

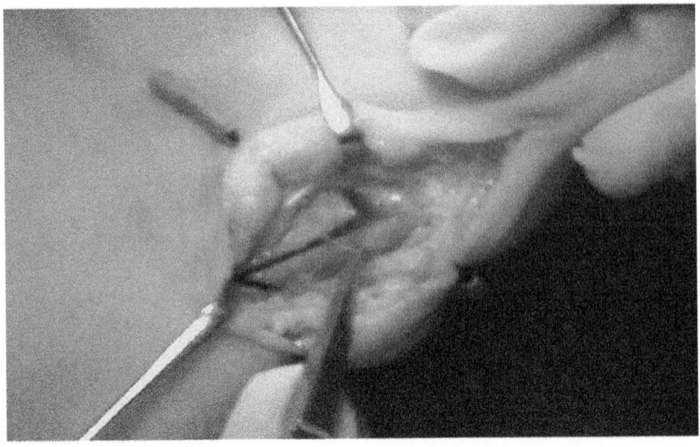

Fig. 2. Short Scafette osteotomy.

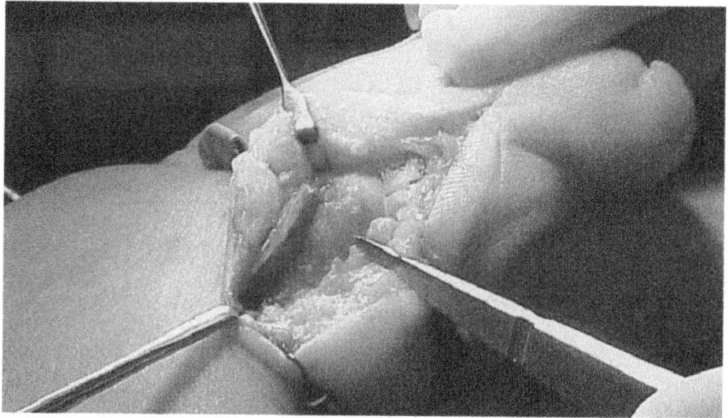

Fig. 3. Short Scarfette osteotomy displaced 5 mm.

averages 4.5°.[2,7] This finding will usually relate to the fifth metatarsal prominence distance (protrusion of the lateral metatarsal head surface from the shaft, measured by a line drawn along the lateral cortex of the fifth metatarsal shaft and another line drawn along the lateral cortex of the fifth metatarsal head; normal, <4 mm)[10]; 4–5

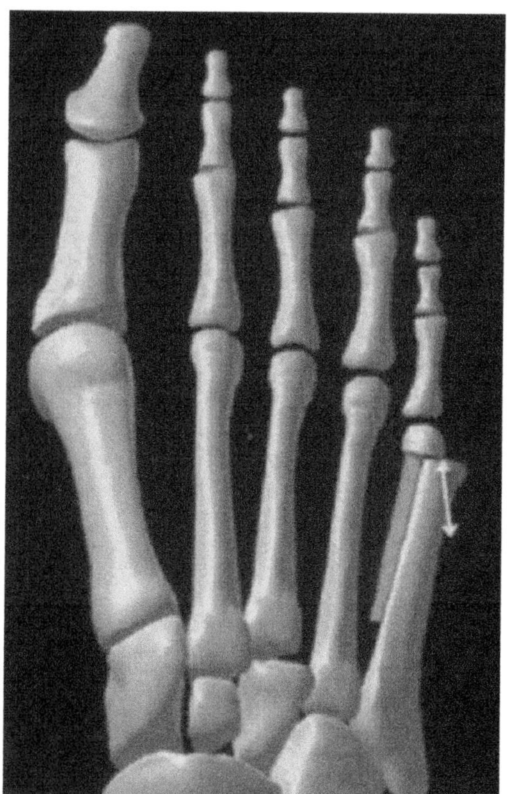

Fig. 4. Long Scarfette osteotomy. Weil 1984 short Scarfette, Barouk 1995 long Scarfette.

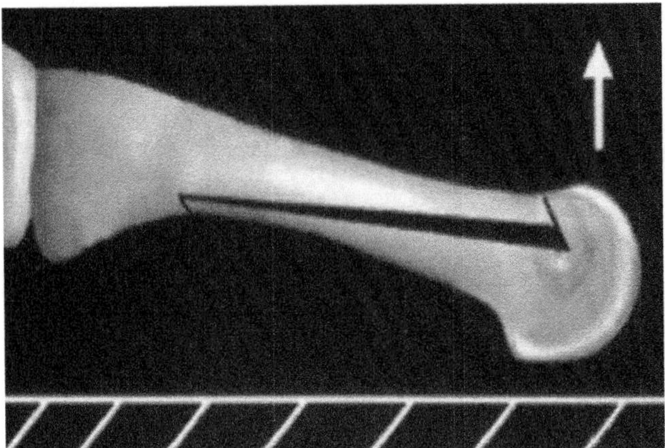

Fig. 5. Long Scarfette osteotomy.

metatarsal head distance (distance between the lateral cortex of the fourth metatarsal head and the medial cortex of the fifth metatarsal head; normal, <3 mm)[11]; and the fifth metatarsal plantar-declination angle (horizontal bisection of the fifth metatarsal in relation to the weight-bearing surface; normal, 108°).[2] The normal length of the fifth

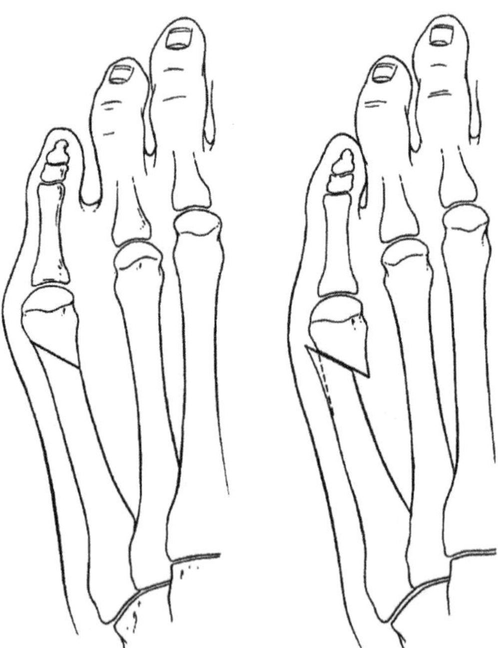

Fig. 6. A medial oblique sliding osteotomy of the fifth metatarsal head using an osteotome to create the osteotomy. This osteotomy was performed through a 1-cm incision overlying the metaphyseal area of the metatarsal area. (*From* Smith SD, Weil LS. Fifth metatarsal osteotomy for tailor's bunion deformity: minor surgery of the foot. Mt. Kiscoe, NY: Futura; 1971; with permission.)

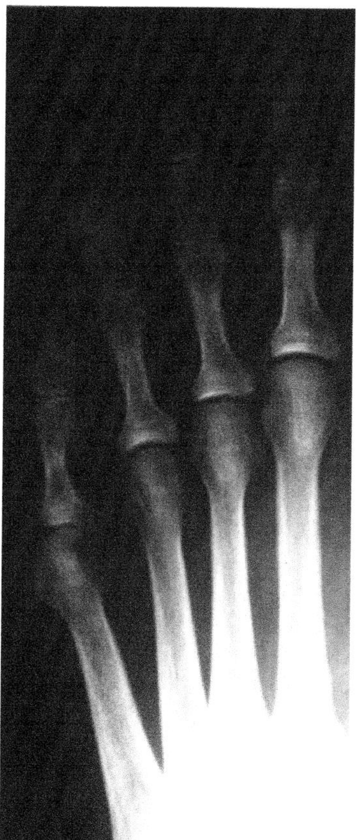

Fig. 7. Giannini's SERI procedure.

metatarsal is considered to be 12 mm shorter than the fourth metatarsal, producing a gentle oblique taper from the central metatarsals in a lateral direction.[2] These findings and observations allow the surgeon to make the determination and selection of the appropriate surgical osteotomy procedure.[2]

One additional observation that should be considered is the position of the bony prominence, keratosis, or "bursitis" on the fifth metatarsal head, namely dorsolateral, lateral, or plantar-lateral? This important finding may influence the decision of which surgical procedure might be best indicated.[9] For example, a plantar keratosis may benefit from a procedure that elevates the metatarsal head along with angular correction; a fifth metatarsal cheilectomy rather than an osteotomy may be appropriate in a case with primarily dorsolateral prominence.

SURGICAL DECISION MAKING FOR BUNIONETTE DEFORMITY

The guidelines for bunionette surgery at the Weil Foot & Ankle Institute are as follows.

In some cases, the prominent dorsal or dorsolateral aspect of the fifth metatarsal head is the symptomatic area and the IMA is normal. In these cases, without large bunionette deformity, a simple dorsolateral cheilectomy is sufficient to alleviate symptoms and an osteotomy is not needed. However, most cases with a bunionette

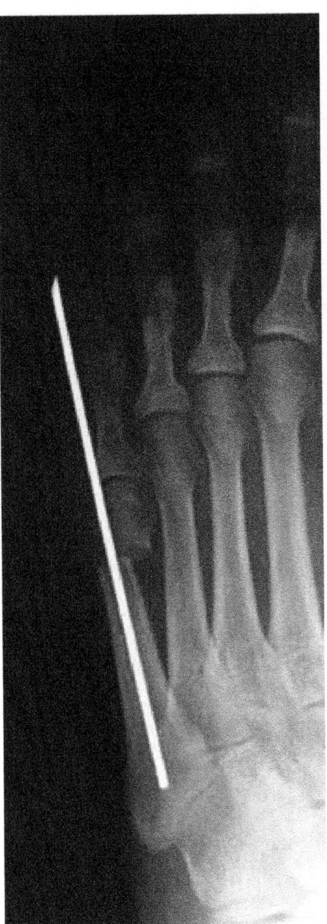

Fig. 8. Giannini's SERI procedure.

demonstrate a 4–5 IMA in excess of 6°. In these cases, an osteotomy is indicated. Our algorithm calls for either a Weil Osteotomy (WO) suggested by Barouk,[15] or a short Scarfette osteotomy with an IMA between 5° and 8°. The WO is commonly recommended because of its inherent stability in the sagittal plane, technical ease, and rapid healing. In the case of an intractable plantar keratosis, a Scarfette osteotomy is the procedure of choice because of its ability to correct the deformity and elevate the head, diminish plantar pressure, and remain stable during healing.

As the IMA and bowing of the fifth metatarsal increase, the Scarfette is carried more proximal, allowing for greater surface area for bony healing and stability (**Figs. 2 and 3**). It is never longer than 50% of the length of the fifth metatarsal and we make it a point to stay away from the proximal meta-diaphyseal region to avoid any potential for non-union in that area.

In cases of a plantar flexed fifth metatarsal head, as seen in a cavus foot, the long Scarfette (**Figs. 4 and 5**) allows for dorsal as well as medial translation to render a more favorable position.

When we encounter a failed case of bunionette correction, we prefer a metatarsal arthroplasty and remove a few millimeters to a full centimeter from the distal articular

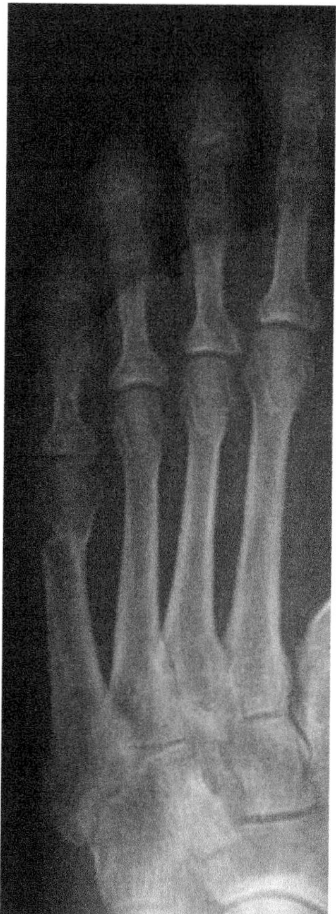

Fig. 9. Giannini's SERI procedure.

surface and perform a plantar condylectomy. This does shorten the toe somewhat, but it is a final correction of the deformity that renders a rapidly healing procedure for a challenging situation.

SURGICAL OSTEOTOMY PROCEDURES

There are many procedures that have been described to correct a bunionette deformity. The following are procedure that will be discussed in this article

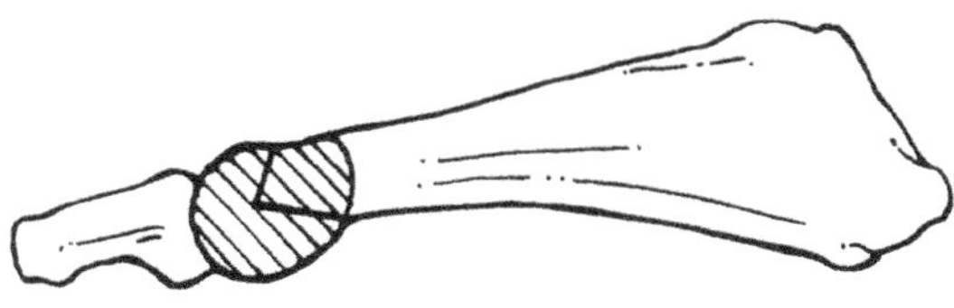

Fig. 10. Chevron osteotomy for bunionette.

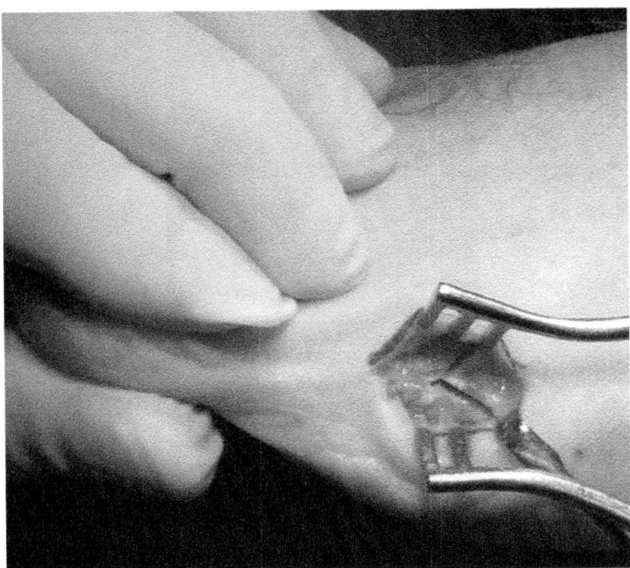

Fig. 11. Intraoperative image of chevron osteotomy.

Medial oblique sliding osteotomy (with fixation)
Medial, oblique slide osteotomy; minimally incision procedure (no fixation) [3,12]
SERI (Giannini—*S*imple, *E*ffective, *R*apid, *I*nexpensive; with fixation)[13]
Chevron (distal osteotomy with or without fixation) [2–4]
Weil osteotomy[15]
Closing, lateral wedge osteotomy at metatarsal neck or proximal diaphysis[2,3,14]
Oblique diaphyseal osteotomy[8]
Scarfette.[3,9,15]

Medial Oblique Sliding Osteotomy

In 1971, Smith and Weil[16] published a technique paper on a medial oblique sliding osteotomy of the fifth metatarsal head using an osteotome to create the osteotomy. This osteotomy was performed through a 1-cm incision overlying the metaphyseal area of the metatarsal area (**Fig. 6**) The 12-mm osteotome was positioned so that an angle was formed of 70° from distal lateral to proximal medial and undercut by 15°. The purpose of this angle was to have the bone slide medially with little chance of lateral subluxation. The undercut of the metatarsal head helped to avoid dorsal migration of the head after surgery. A dressing was applied, bandaging the fifth toe in an abducted position to ensure medialization of the metatarsal head. Patients were advised to maintain guarded weight bearing for 1 week. The results were good with respect to ultimate cosmetic appearance but chronic swelling and 3 to 4 months of healing were necessary for complete resolution.

Minimal Incision Surgery

Bunionette correction via an osteotomy through a minimal incision may be performed using several methods. Probber and White[12] popularized the procedure. Under a local anesthetic, a puncture incision was made at the lateral metaphysis of the flare

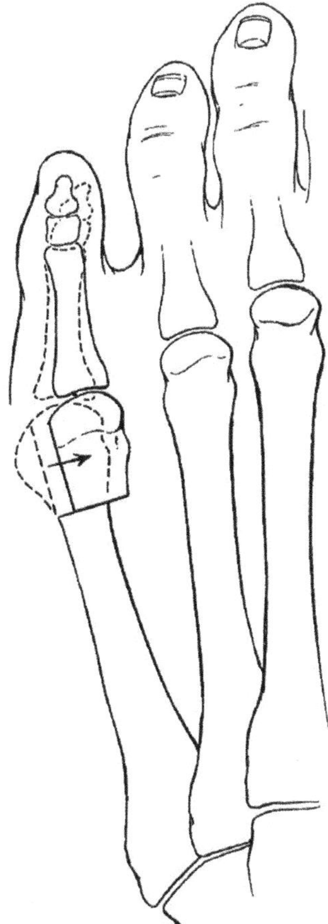

Fig. 12. Medial translation of the distal fragment correction.

of the fifth metatarsal head.[12] A "dental cutting burr" was used to create a "blind" osteotomy at a 90° angle to the metatarsal shaft. Some minimal incision surgeons used fluoroscopy to verify the intraoperative position. The cut allowed for mobilization of the fifth metatarsal head in a medial direction to correct the deformity. The bone debris (paste) caused by the high-torque–low-speed burr was extirpated out through the dermal opening and the wound irrigated and closed with a single 0.25-in.

Steri-strip. No fixation was utilized and a compression dressing was applied, bandaging the fifth toe in an abducted position to ensure medialization of the metatarsal head. Patients were permitted to ambulate immediately and return to work as needed. Retrospective, uncontrolled results of the procedure were published with relatively short-term follow-ups. However, personal observations of our senior author (LSW) were remarkably good with respect to clinical outcome but with a high complication rate. Wound problems caused by the heat of the rotary burr usually healed uneventfully but some became infected. Chronic swelling lasting up to 3 to 5 months was not infrequent with this unfixed osteotomy. Non-union was infrequent, perhaps because the bone paste caused by the rotary burr facilitated healing of the osteotomy. Uncontrolled, dorsal elevation was observed that led to metatarsalgia

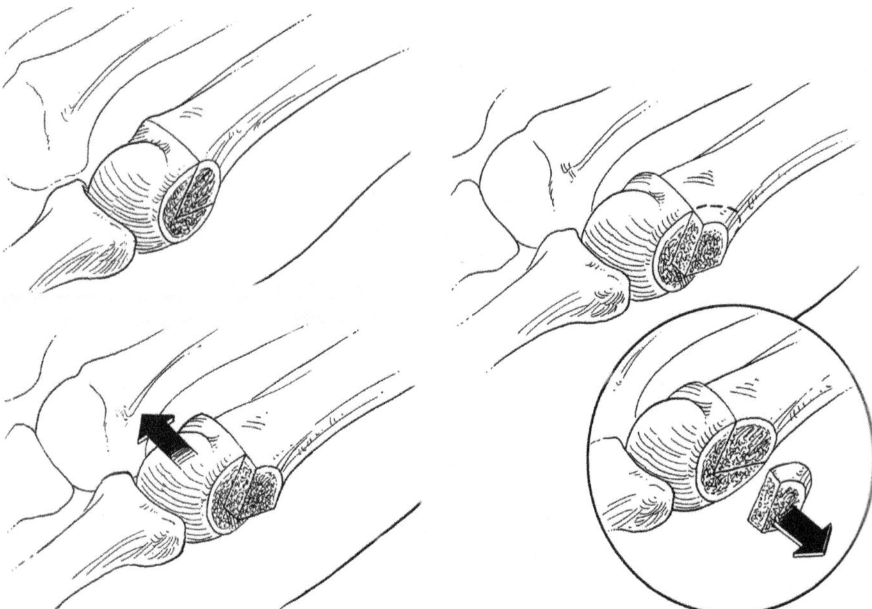

Fig. 13. Chevron osteotomy. (*From* Throckmorton JK, Bradlee N. Transverse V sliding osteotomy: A new surgical procedure for the correction of Tailor's bunion deformity. J Foot Surg 1978;18:117–21; with permission.)

under the fourth metatarsal head and this appeared to be the most adverse complication that needed revision surgery. The great majority of cases yielded an acceptable cosmetic result with no scarring or dorsal contracture. The procedure has recently become popular with orthopedic surgeons in Spain, France, and Italy. Because of the limited outcomes studies available and the tendency toward dorsal malunion, however, it is difficult to recommend this technique routinely until more extensive data are reported.

An alternative mini-incision technique utilizing fixation was reported by Giannini and colleagues[13] (**Fig. 7**). A 1-cm lateral incision is made just proximal to the lateral eminence of the fifth metatarsal head through the skin and subcutaneous tissue, down to bone. Once the lateral aspect of the metatarsal neck is visualized, the osteotomy is performed. The inclination of the osteotomy in the lateral-to-medial direction is perpendicular to the fourth ray if the length of the fifth metatarsal bone is to be maintained. The osteotomy is inclined in a distal–proximal direction up to 25°, if shortening of the metatarsal bone or decompression of the metatarsophalangeal joint is desired in cases of mild joint arthritis. More rarely, if a lengthening of the fifth metatarsal bone was necessary, the osteotomy is inclined in a proximal–distal direction up to 15°.

After creation of the osteotomy with the saw, the head is mobilized with a small osteotome and medial translation of the metatarsal head is performed, introducing the Kirschner wire superficial to the lateral eminence. Plantar translation of the metatarsal head, if desired, is produced by introducing the Kirschner wire in the upper aspect of the metatarsal head. A 1.8-mm Kirschner wire is inserted into the soft tissue adjacent to the bone in a proximal-to-distal direction along the longitudinal axis of the fifth toe. The Kirschner wire exits at the lateral area of the tip of the toe, adjacent to

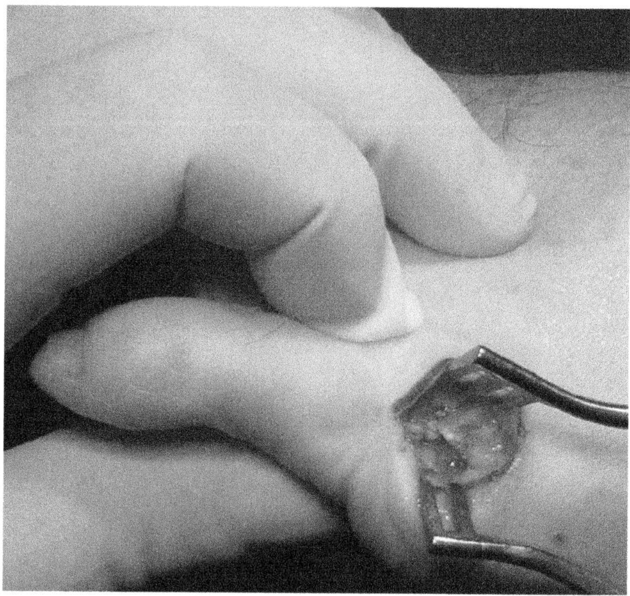

Fig. 14. Manual translation and impact of head on shaft.

the lateral border of the nail; it is retracted with the drill up to the proximal end of the osteotomy. The metatarsal head is then translated medially and the Kirschner wire is advanced retrograde into the diaphyseal canal toward the metatarsal base (**Fig. 8**). If the cut edge of the metatarsal is laterally prominent, a small wedge of bone is removed. The skin is sutured with a single 3-0 stitch. The Kirschner wire is bent and cut at the tip of the toe. Ambulation is allowed immediately using a postoperative shoe that allows weight bearing only on the hind foot. After 1 month, the dressing, suture, and Kirschner wire are removed (**Fig. 9**). Patients are allowed to return to normal comfortable shoe wear, while gentle exercises with cycling and swimming are advised.

Giannini and colleagues reported that 48 of 50 patients were satisfied with their result. The preoperative American Orthopedic Foot and Ankle Society (AOFAS) forefoot score was 62.8 ± 15.1 points (range, 19–80) and postoperatively it was 94 ± 6.8 points (range, 75–100) ($P<.0005$). Thirty-eight (76%) feet were rated as excellent, 9 (18%) good, 2 (4%) fair, and 1 (2%) was considered poor. Pain was absent in 40 (80%) feet, mild or occasional in 8 (16%) feet, and moderate or daily in 2 (4%) feet. Function in 42 (84%) feet had no limitations in daily and sport activities, 7 (14%) had minimal limitations, and 1 (2%) foot had a severe limitation. Forty-four (88%) patients were able to wear normal shoes.

All osteotomies healed radiographically at an average of 3 months. All the osteotomies remodeled over time, even in cases with significant offset initially. Radiographic evaluation demonstrated that the average fifth MTP angle was 16.8° ± 5.1° preoperatively and 7.9° ± 3.1° ($P<.0005$) postoperatively. The 4–5 IMA was 12° ± 1.7° preoperatively and 6.7° ± 1.7° postoperatively ($P<.0005$). No severe complications, such as avascular necrosis of the metatarsal head or non-union of the osteotomy, occurred. In 6 (12%) feet, the radiographic healing of the osteotomy occurred over 4 months after surgery; however, no increased postoperative pain was

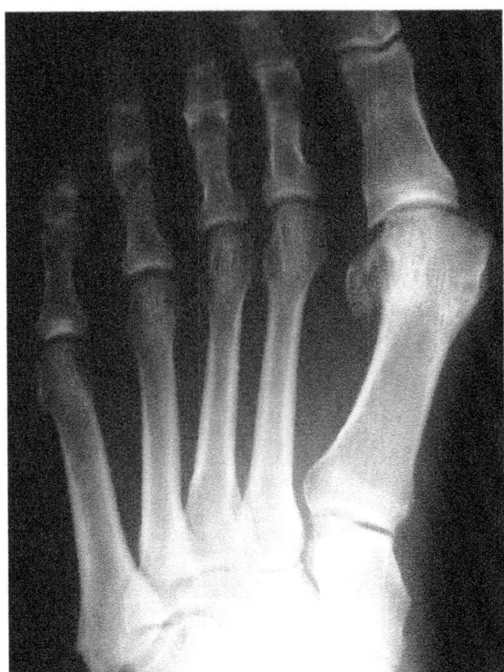

Fig. 15. Preoperative image of bunionette.

noted in these patients, nor was the clinical result compromised at final follow-up. Further, no correlation was found between the delayed radiographic union and the offset at the osteotomy; in fact, none of these cases displaced. One (2%) foot had a skin inflammatory reaction around the Kirschner wire. Two (4%) feet reported symptomatic plantar callosities under the fourth metatarsal heads. No dorsal subluxation of the fifth metatarsophalangeal joint (MTPJ) was present. Further studies with larger numbers of patients, longer follow-up, determination of the risk of dorsal malunion or metatarsalgia, and stratification for severity of deformity are necessary before recommending this procedure on a widespread basis.

Chevron Osteotomy

Following the success of a stable construct for the Austin (chevron) hallux bunionectomy, several authors,[2] including Kitaoka,[4] utilized a similar technique for the bunionette deformity.

Through a dorsal or lateral incision, a lateral exostectomy was performed on the fifth metatarsal head, removing a small amount of bone. A chevron osteotomy was then performed in the cancellous bone of the metatarsal head (**Figs. 10 and 11**). The head was mobilized and translated medially by about 3 to 6 mm (**Figs. 12 and 13**). Using manual compression the fifth metatarsal head was firmly compressed from distal to proximal (**Fig. 14**). The lateral overhanging ledge that remained was carefully resected so as to not interrupt the osteotomy position. Later, some surgeons chose to use fixation with a K-wire to avoid malunion and delayed healing (**Figs. 15 and 16**). Currently, surgeons routinely use absorbable pins or small-diameter screws for fixation (**Fig. 17**). Guarded weight bearing was recommended and most patients had

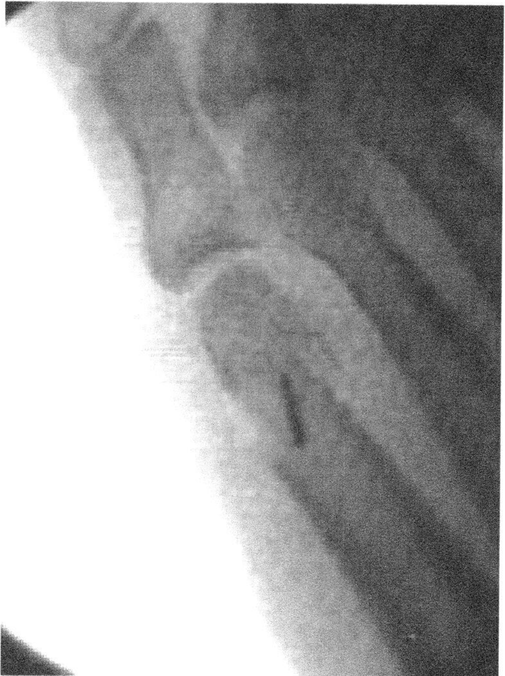

Fig. 16. Intraoperative fluoroscopic image of chevron with pin fixation.

a very favorable outcome. Healing usually took 2 to 3 months for resolution of swelling and the cosmetic appearance was good. However, in larger deformities with a 4–5 IMA >8° to 10°, the width of the fifth metatarsal head just did not allow enough medial displacement to reduce the deformity adequately. As such, this may be a good option for smaller deformities or cases with outflaring of the distal metatarsal shaft that do not require as large a correction.

Weil Metatarsal Osteotomy

Another option is the oblique sliding metatarsal osteotomy (or Weil osteotomy) commonly performed on the central metatarsals for correction of clawtoes or metatarsalgia. An osteotomy is created from the dorsum of the metatarsal head–neck junction heading plantarward parallel to the plantar surface of the foot. The metatarsal head is then translated medially to reduce the IMA and fixed with a dorsal-to-plantar twist-off or solid lag screw. The lateral overhanging bone and lateral eminence are trimmed off. Barouk[15] recommends the Weil osteotomy for small to intermediate deformities because of its inherent stability and ease of performing this procedure (**Fig. 18**). However, like the chevron procedure, it has limitations in the narrow metatarsal head; in such cases, the distal fragment can be translated only a small amount to still have sufficient bony apposition for fixation and healing. Literature reports on the use of this osteotomy for correction of the bunionette deformity are sparse, but the senior author (LSW) has extensive personal experience with its use and has found it to produce good clinical outcomes with a reproducible technique.

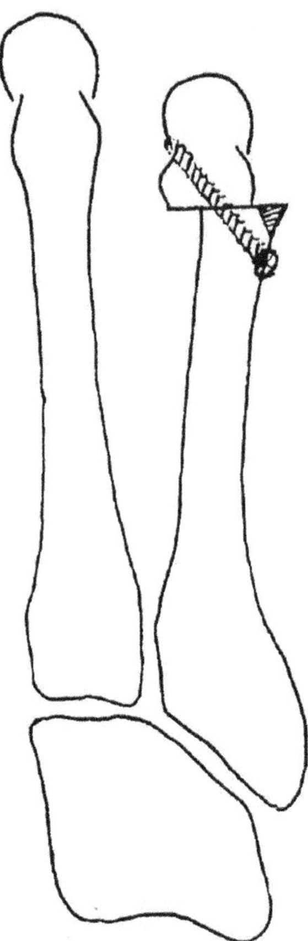

Fig. 17. Small diameter screw for fixation. (*From* Frankel JP, Turf RM, King BA. Tailor's bunion: clinical evaluation and correction by distal metaphyseal osteotomy with cortical screw fixation. J Foot Surg 1989;28:237–43; with permission.)

Proximal Closing Wedge Osteotomy

In cases of a severely widened 4–5 IMA, distal osteotomies have insufficient power for correction and a more powerful proximal osteotomy is preferred. In 1972, Gerbert and colleagues[14] presented preliminary results of a fifth metatarsal shaft osteotomy described as a long oblique wedge resection.

A dorsal incision measuring 4 to 5 cm in length is placed directly overlying the fifth metatarsal neck and shaft from the fifth metatarsal to the junction between the proximal and middle one third of the fifth metatarsal. The incision is deepened directly through the skin to the level of the capsule and periosteum overlying the fifth metatarsal neck and shaft. A long oblique osteotomy was outlined from distal–medial to proximal–lateral and terminating at the junction of the lateral shaft and base of the fifth metatarsal. The osteotomy was performed in such a manner as to maintain the proximal–lateral cortical–periosteal hinge. A small 2- to 3-mm medially based wedge of bone was then resected from the proximal and medial portion of the fifth metatarsal and the proximal–lateral hinge gently "feathered" as described previously (**Figs. 19–21**). A small bone clamp is used to close the osteotomy, which rotates the distal

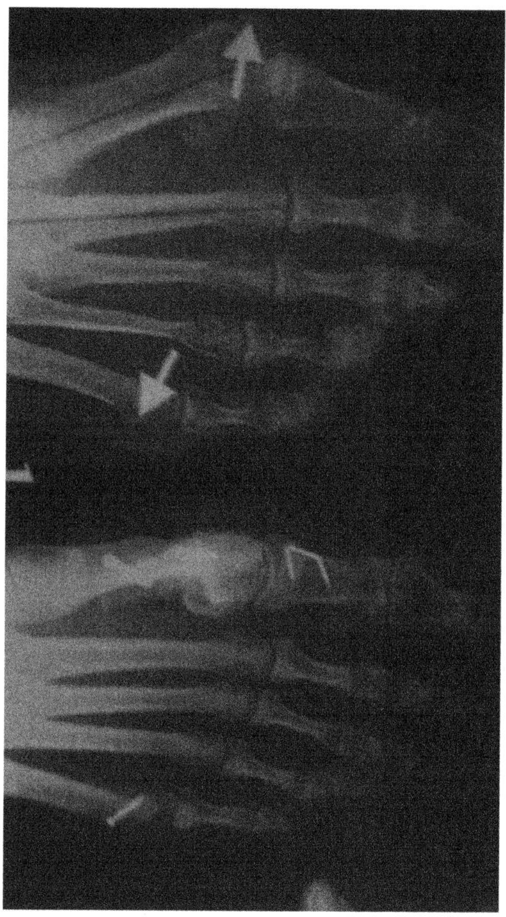

Fig. 18. Preoperative and postoperative Weil osteotomy of the fifth metatarsal for bunionette.

fifth metatarsal, capital fragment medially. If any gapping is present between the distal and proximal capital fragments, reciprocal planing is used or the small wedge of bone resected then morselized and packed within the gap as a bone graft. Fluoroscopy is used to verify complete reduction of the deformity before performing final fixation with a small, oblique screw, oriented from distal–lateral to proximal–medial at the junction between the osteotomy and the fifth metatarsal shaft. The fifth digit is bandaged in a slightly overcorrected and abducted and plantarflexed position. This technique does not allow for immediate weight bearing because of the orientation and fragility of the osteotomy and, therefore, should be protected non–weight-bearing in either a short-leg cast or removable immobilization boot. Serial radiographs are obtained to monitor osseous healing and, once verified, the patient is allowed to return to a roomy athletic or oxford shoe with weight bearing to tolerance. This can occur from 6 to 8 weeks. Castle and colleagues,[17] in a retrospective review of 26 long oblique wedge resection osteotomies, found a mean 4–5 IMA reduction of 1.58 (7.9–6.48) and a mean lateral deviation angle reduction of 3.98 (4.1–0.28). One osteotomy fractured after a traumatic incident in the early postoperative period but there were no reported

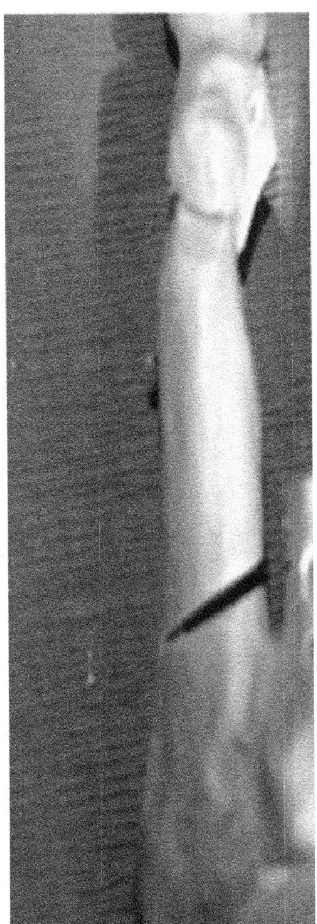

Fig. 19. Closing medial wedge at neck and oblique shaft osteotomy for bunionette deformity.

incidences of delayed union, malunion, or transfer lesions. This osteotomy appears most useful for the correction of an abnormally large 4–5 IMA.

Oblique Diaphyseal Osteotomy

Coughlin described an oblique mid-shaft osteotomy to correct an increases 4–5 IMA and/or an increased lateral bowing[2,8] (**Fig. 22**). This oblique osteotomy is rotational rather than translational, which helps to maintain metatarsal length and avoid shortening. A lateral incision is created over the fifth metatarsal shaft and MTPJ. A capsulotomy is performed at the joint and the lateral eminence resected. Before the osteotomy, a proximal drill hole can be created for placement of a small diameter lag screw. The oblique osteotomy is created with the saw from dorsal–proximal to plantar–distal with the saw perpendicular to the shaft. The distal fragment can then be rotated using the screw as a hinge, thereby reducing the IMA (**Figs. 23 and 24**). A second screw is then inserted to stabilize the construct. Imbrication of the lateral MTP capsule then corrects toe alignment to complete the procedure. In cases with a plantar keratosis, the saw blade can be inclined slightly cephalad rather than perpendicular to the diaphysis; when the osteotomy is rotated, this will slightly elevate the metatarsal head and unload the area of the callus.

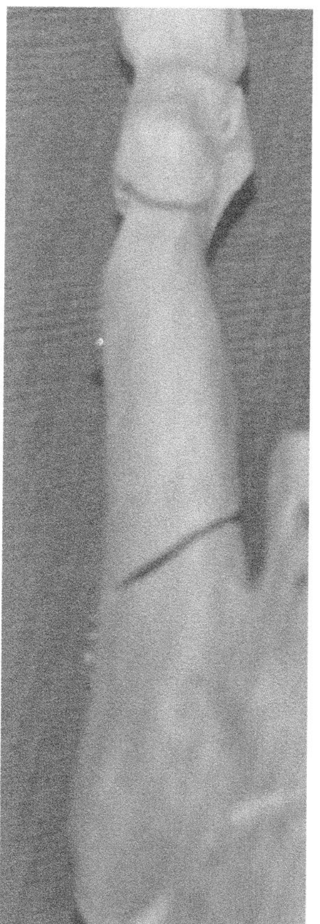

Fig. 20. Closing medial wedge at neck and oblique shaft osteotomy for bunionette deformity.

Coughlin[8] reported a series of 30 feet (20 patients) who underwent this procedure with 31 months follow-up. Ninety-three percent had excellent or good clinical results. The mean 4–5 IMA corrected from 10.6° preoperatively to 0.8° postoperatively. All osteotomies healed within 8 weeks, with only one case of a mild transfer lesion. He concluded that internal fixation led to high rates of healing with low complications. These findings were reproduced in another series by Vienne and coworkers.[18] In this series, 33 patients were followed prospectively after oblique diaphyseal osteotomy for 24 months. Ninety-one percent had excellent or good clinical outcomes, with similar radiographic correction to Coughlin's original series. They noted no instances of delayed union or non-union. Both series did note a relatively high rate of the need for hardware removal, likely due to the subcutaneous position of the fifth metatarsal and screws.

Scarfette Osteotomy

Based on the favorable results of the Scarf procedure for hallux valgus deformity, Weil proposed a "reverse scarf procedure" for the bunionette deformity.[9] Barouk later popularized the procedure and gave it the name Scarfette.[15] The 3-cm, laterally

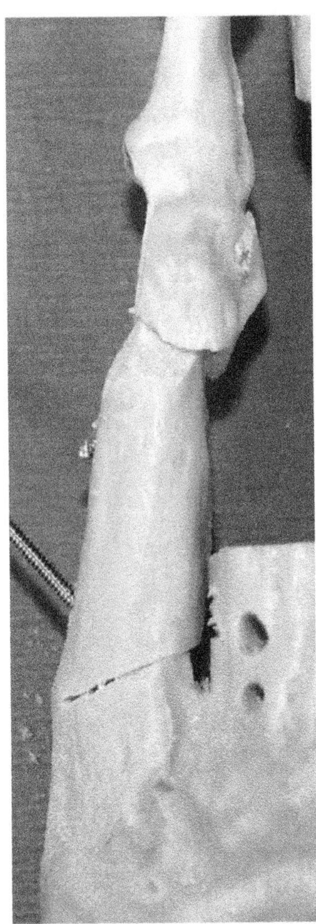

Fig. 21. Closing medial wedge at neck and oblique shaft osteotomy for bunionette deformity.

based incision is carried directly through the capsule and periosteum which are sharply reflected to expose the dorsal and plantar lateral aspects of the fifth metatarsal head and neck. A minimal lateral exostectomy is performed with a power saw. The scarf-shaped cut, about 2.5 cm long, is outlined from dorsal distal to plantar proximal on the fifth metatarsal head and neck (**Fig. 25**). A 60° dorsal–distal osteotomy is performed 3 mm proximal to the articular cartilage of the fifth metatarsal head. Next, the central horizontal osteotomy directed from superior to inferior is performed with the saw held in slight dorsal angulation so as not to plantar displace the osteotomy fragment. Lastly, a proximal 60° plantar osteotomy is performed at the proximal plantar extent of the horizontal osteotomy (see **Fig. 25**).

The neck of the fifth metatarsal shaft bows plantarly, so it is important to note that the proximal portion of the osteotomy does not end up at mid-shaft. It should be at the plantar 1/3 of the metatarsal shaft to avoid potential stress fracture. A small, thin osteotome is inserted in the osteotomy and gently rotated to verify completion of the osteotomy. With traction on the fifth digit, the fifth metatarsal head is gently manipulated in a medial direction to reduce the deformity. Once completed, a small clamp is placed on the lateral fifth metatarsal shaft and the osteotomy fragment. Fixation was initially performed with manual impaction and capsulorraphy but

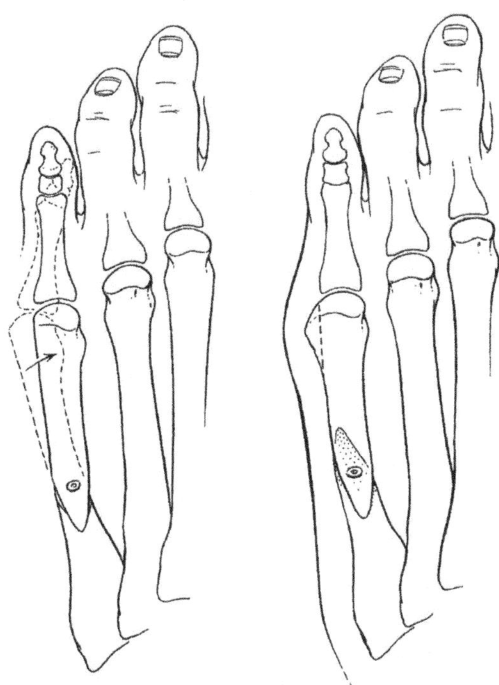

Fig. 22. Oblique diaphyseal osteotomy. (*From* Coughlin MJ. Correction of the bunionette with midshaft oblique osteotomy. Orthopedic Trans 1998;12:30–1; with permission.)

some cases developed displacement, so fixation with a buried threaded 1.6-mm pin or 2.5 mm screw was used thereafter. Once adequate correction is obtained, the osteotomy fragment is impacted on the metatarsal (**Fig. 26**). The remaining lateral head, neck, and shaft are carefully removed and smoothed with power instrumentation (**Fig. 27**). The periosteum and capsule are repaired with 3-0 absorbable suture. A running subcuticular stitch followed by Steri-strips are used to repair the skin. The postoperative period was standard for each patient. This included a bulky dressing with the fifth toe bandaged in abduction and a surgical shoe with patients using guarded weight bearing, immediately after surgery. At the first postoperative appointment 1 week later, all patients were transitioned into a running shoe and started physical therapy for strengthening and range-of-motion exercises.

Follow-up was performed in 50 patients at an average of 12 months.[19] The average age was 50.23 ± 14.31 years. There were 44 (88%) females and 6 (1.2%) males. The operative side included 27(54%) right and 23 (46%) left feet. Preoperatively the mean 4–5 IMA, LDA, and fifth MTPJ angles were 10.34° ± 2.40°, 4.15° ± 4.08°, and 15.56° ± 6.83°, respectively. Nineteen (38%) patients had a type 2 deformity and 31 (62%) patients had a type 3 deformity. The 19 patients with a type 2 deformity had a mean LDA of 9.0° ± 3.46°. Postoperatively at 1 year, the mean 4–5 IMA, LDA, and fifth MTPJ angles were corrected to 1.80° ± 2.21°, 0.24° ± 0.46°, and 2.40° ± 7.94°, respectively. Postoperative correction of the 4–5 IMA, LDA, and fifth MTPJ angles were statistically significant ($P<.001$). Complications included one undercorrection and seven hardware removals.

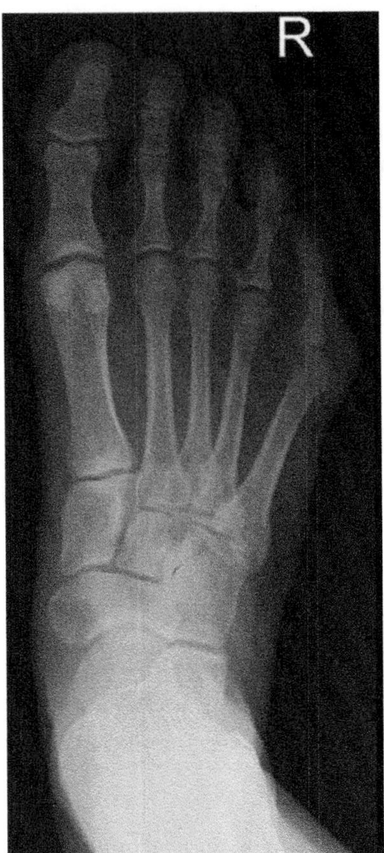

Fig. 23. Preoperative oblique mid-shaft Coughlin osteotomy.

Kilmartin[20] reported on 63 patients who underwent operative repair of 77 tailor's bunion deformities with a Scarfette technique between September 1999 and September 2006. Eighty-six percent were completely satisfied, 11.4% were satisfied with reservations, and 3% were dissatisfied. Ninety-one percent considered themselves better than before their surgery whereas 8.6% felt they were no better. Ninety-one percent of patients said they would undergo surgery under the same conditions again. Preoperatively, the mean 4–5 IMA measured on weight bearing radiographs was 9.9° (SD, 2.2) and the mean postoperative IMA was 5.7° (SD, 2.0). The mean preoperative AOFAS score was 44.1 points (SD, 14.5) and the mean postoperative score at 6-month review was 91.8 (SD, 20.2). The clinical improvement was maintained, with the AOFAS score at final review 36 months of 88.1 (SD, 11.6).

SUMMARY

A variety of surgical osteotomy procedures have been described for the bunionette deformity.

Metatarsal osteotomies narrow the forefoot, maintain the length of the metatarsal, and preserve function of the metatarsophalangeal joint. Distal metatarsal osteotomies produce less correction and reduce postoperative disability; however, they pose a

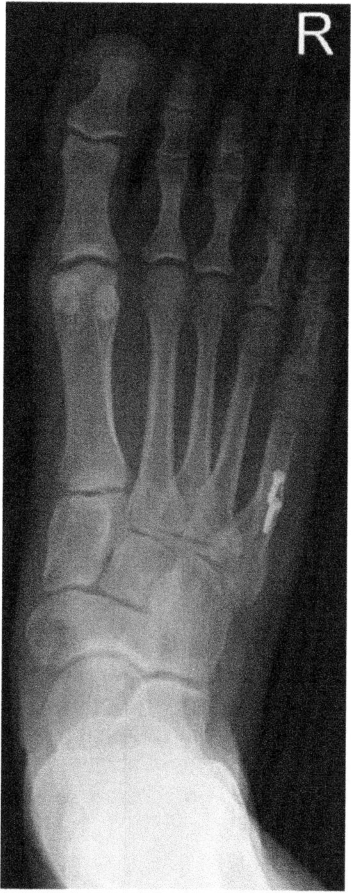

Fig. 24. Postoperative oblique mid-shaft Coughlin osteotomy.

risk of inadequate correction because of the small width of the fifth metatarsal head and transfer lesions if shortened or dorsiflexed excessively. The sliding oblique metaphyseal osteotomy described by Smith and Weil (without fixation) and later by Steinke[21] (with fixation) is easy to perform and provides good cancellous bone contact. Fixation is sometimes difficult and bone healing can take a few months owing to the unstable construct of this osteotomy. Kitaoka described a distal chevron osteotomy, which provides lateral pressure relief and reduced plantar pressure.[4] This osteotomy is currently the most common procedure used; however, it may prove difficult to perform if the deformity is large and the bone is narrow. Diaphyseal osteotomies are indicated when greater correction is needed; however, they require more dissection and there is greater postoperative convalescence with non–weight bearing for several weeks. Proximal base osteotomies may be used to address significantly increased 4–5 IMAs or when a large degree of sagittal plane correction is required. Approaches that have been described include opening and closing base wedges and basal chevrons. Advantages to this approach are the ability to avoid epiphyseal plates in pediatric patients and maintain function of the MTPJ, while disadvantages include inherent instability of the location of the

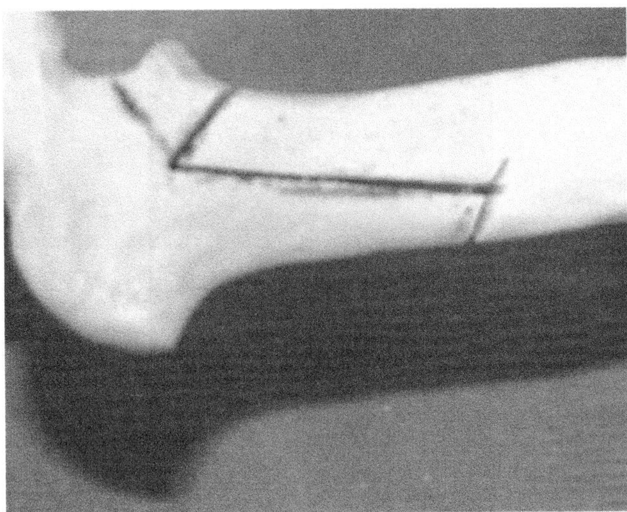

Fig. 25. Scarfette cut for bunionette. Note the proximal **low** cut.

osteotomy, embarrassment of intraosseous and extraosseus blood supply of the metatarsal, and technical demand. Non–weight bearing is essential for several weeks. The Scarfette procedure is a combination head–shaft procedure, which is indicated to treat mild to moderate transverse and sagittal plane deformities.[9,19] The inherent stability of the osteotomy and ability for early weight bearing of the Scarfette makes this our procedure of choice when selecting treatments for patients with a bunionette deformity.

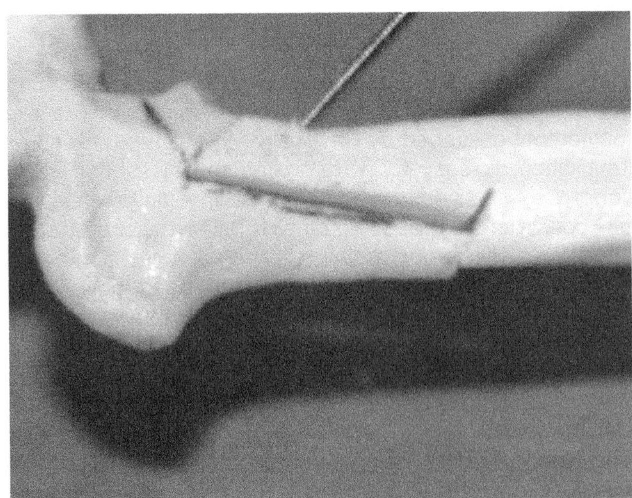

Fig. 26. Distal fragment displaced medially, then impacted and fixed with threaded pin or screw.

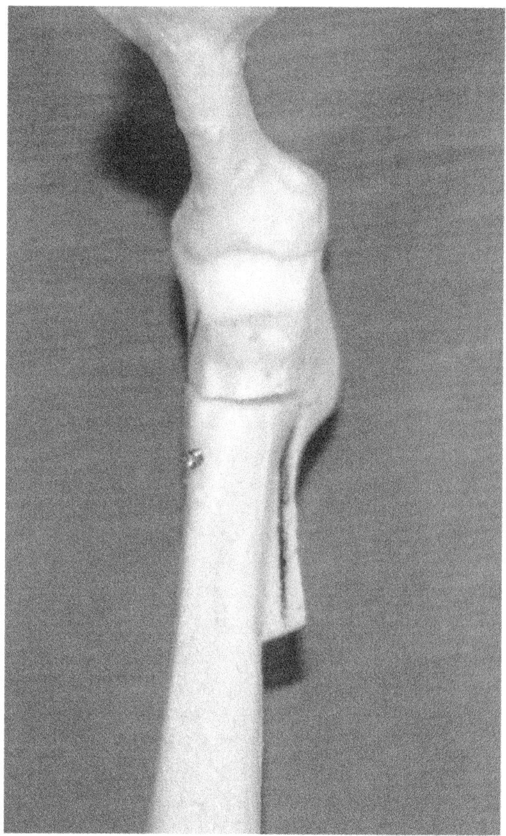

Fig. 27. Scarfette displacement with very stable construct.

ACKNOWLEDGMENTS

The authors express a special thank you to Thomas Roukis, DPM, for his help with illustrations and photos.

REFERENCES

1. Davies H. Metatarsus quintus valgus. Br Med J 1949;1:664–5.
2. American College of Foot and Ankle Surgeons. Tailor's bunion and associated fifth metatarsal conditions: preferred practice guidelines. Park Ridge (IL): American College of Foot and Ankle Surgeons; 1993.
3. Roukis TS. The tailor's bunionette deformity: a field guide to surgical correction. Clin Podiatr Med Surg 2005;22(2):223–45.
4. Kitaoka HB, Holiday AD Jr. Lateralcondyl ar resection for bunionette. Clin Orthop 1992;278:183–92.
5. Diebold PF. Basal osteotomy of the fifth metatarsal for bunionette. J.Foot Ankle 1991;12:74–79.
6. Hansson G. Sliding osteotomy for tailor's bunion: brief report. J Bone Joint Surg (Br) 1989; 71(2):324.
7. Fallat LM, Bucholz J. Analysis of the tailor's bunion by radiographic and anatomic display. J Am Podiatr Assoc 1980;70(12):597–603.

8. Coughlin MJ. Treatment of bunionette deformity with longitudinal diaphyseal osteotomy with distal soft tissue repair. Foot Ankle 1991;11:195–203.
9. Weil LS. The reverse scarf osteotomy for tailor bunion deformity. Seoul (South Korea): SICOT; 1992.
10. Karasick D. Preoperative assessment of symptomatic bunionette deformity: radiologic findings. Am J Radiol 1995;164(1):147–9.
11. Nestor BJ, Kitaoka HB, Ilstrup DM, et al. Radiologic anatomy of the painful bunionette. Foot Ankle 1990;11:6 –11.
12. White DL. Minimal incision approach to osteotomies of the lesser metatarsals: for treatment of intractable keratosis, metatarsalgia, and tailor's bunion. Clin Podiatr Med Surg 1991;8(1):25–9.
13. Giannini S, Faldini C, Vannini F, et al. The minimally invasive osteotomy "S.E.R.I." (Simple, Effective, Rapid, Inexpensive) for correction of bunionette deformity. Foot Ankle Int 2008;29(3):282–6.
14. Gerbert J, Sgarlato TE, Subotnick SI. Preliminary study of a closing wedge osteotomy of the fifth metatarsal for correction of a tailor's bunion deformity. J Am Podiatr Assoc 972;62(6):212– 8.
15. Barouk LS. Some pathologies of the fifth ray: tailor's bunion. In: Barouk LS, editor. Forefoot reconstruction. Paris: Springer-Verlag; 2002. p. 276–83.
16. Smith SD, Weil LS. Fifth metatarsal osteotomy for tailor's bunion deformity: minor surgery of the foot. Mt. Kiscoe, NY: Futura; 1971.
17. Castle JE, Cohen AH, Docks G. Fifth metatarsal distal oblique wedge osteotomy utilizing cortical screw fixation. J Foot Surg 1992;31(5):478–85.
18. Vienne P, Oesselmann M, Espinosa N, et al. Modified Coughlin procedure for surgical treatment of symptomatic tailor's bunion: a prospective followup study of 33 consecutive operations. Foot Ankle Int 2006;27(8):573–80.
19. Glover J, Weil L Jr, Weil L Sr. Scarfette osteotomy for surgical treatment of bunionette deformity. Foot Ankle Spec 2009;2(2):73–8.
20. Maher AJ, Kilmartin TE. Scarf osteotomy for correction of tailor's bunion: mid- to long-term followup. Foot Ankle Int 2010;31(8):676–82.
21. Steinke MS, Boll KL. Hohmann-Thomasen metatarsal osteotomy for tailor's bunion (bunionette). J Bone Joint Surg (Am) 1989;71(3):423–6.

Index

Note: Page numbers of article titles are in **boldface** type.

Foot Ankle Clin N Am 16 (2011) 713–721
doi:10.1016/S1083-7515(11)00088-X

E

F

G

H

I

J

K

L

M

United States Postal Service

Statement of Ownership, Management, and Circulation (All Periodicals Publications Except Requestor Publications)

1. Publication Title: Foot and Ankle Clinics
2. Publication Number: 0 1 6 - 3 6 8
3. Filing Date: 9/16/11
4. Issue Frequency: Mar, Jun, Sep, Dec
5. Number of Issues Published Annually: 4
6. Annual Subscription Price: $271.00
7. Complete Mailing Address of Known Office of Publication (*Not printer*) (*Street, city, county, state, and ZIP+4®*)

   Elsevier Inc.
   360 Park Avenue South
   New York, NY 10010-1710

   Contact Person: Stephen Bushing
   Telephone (Include area code): 215-239-3688

8. Complete Mailing Address of Headquarters or General Business Office of Publisher (*Not printer*)

   Elsevier Inc., 360 Park Avenue South, New York, NY 10010-1710

9. Full Names and Complete Mailing Addresses of Publisher, Editor, and Managing Editor (*Do not leave blank*)

   Publisher (*Name and complete mailing address*)
   Kim Murphy, Elsevier, Inc., 1600 John F. Kennedy Blvd. Suite 1800, Philadelphia, PA 19103-2899

   Editor (*Name and complete mailing address*)
   David Parsons, Elsevier, Inc., 1600 John F. Kennedy Blvd. Suite 1800, Philadelphia, PA 19103-2899

   Managing Editor (*Name and complete mailing address*)
   Barbara Cohen-Kligerman, Elsevier, Inc., 1600 John F. Kennedy Blvd. Suite 1800, Philadelphia, PA 19103-2899

10. Owner (*Do not leave blank. If the publication is owned by a corporation, give the name and address of the corporation immediately followed by the names and addresses of all stockholders owning or holding 1 percent or more of the total amount of stock. If not owned by a corporation, give the names and addresses of the individual owners. If owned by a partnership or other unincorporated firm, give its name and address as well as those of each individual owner. If the publication is published by a nonprofit organization, give its name and address.*)

Full Name	Complete Mailing Address
Wholly owned subsidiary of	4520 East-West Highway
Reed/Elsevier, US holdings	Bethesda, MD 20814

11. Known Bondholders, Mortgagees, and Other Security Holders Owning or Holding 1 Percent or More of Total Amount of Bonds, Mortgages, or Other Securities. If none, check box → ☐ None

Full Name	Complete Mailing Address
N/A	

12. Tax Status (*For completion by nonprofit organizations authorized to mail at nonprofit rates*) (*Check one*)
    The purpose, function, and nonprofit status of this organization and the exempt status for federal income tax purposes:
    ☐ Has Not Changed During Preceding 12 Months
    ☐ Has Changed During Preceding 12 Months (*Publisher must submit explanation of change with this statement*)

PS Form **3526**, September 2007 (Page 1 of 3 (Instructions Page 3)) PSN 7530-01-000-9931 **PRIVACY NOTICE**: See our Privacy policy in www.usps.com

13. Publication Title: Foot and Ankle Clinics
14. Issue Date for Circulation Data Below: June 2011

15. Extent and Nature of Circulation		Average No. Copies Each Issue During Preceding 12 Months	No. Copies of Single Issue Published Nearest to Filing Date
a. Total Number of Copies (*Net press run*)		1340	1320
b. Paid Circulation (By Mail and Outside the Mail)	(1) Mailed Outside-County Paid Subscriptions Stated on PS Form 3541. (*Include paid distribution above nominal rate, advertiser's proof copies, and exchange copies*)	716	651
	(2) Mailed In-County Paid Subscriptions Stated on PS Form 3541 (*Include paid distribution above nominal rate, advertiser's proof copies, and exchange copies*)		
	(3) Paid Distribution Outside the Mails Including Sales Through Dealers and Carriers, Street Vendors, Counter Sales, and Other Paid Distribution Outside USPS®	150	121
	(4) Paid Distribution by Other Classes Mailed Through the USPS (e.g. First-Class Mail®)		
c. Total Paid Distribution (*Sum of 15b (1), (2), (3), and (4)*) ►		866	772
d. Free or Nominal Rate Distribution (By Mail and Outside the Mail)	(1) Free or Nominal Rate Outside-County Copies Included on PS Form 3541	40	46
	(2) Free or Nominal Rate In-County Copies Included on PS Form 3541		
	(3) Free or Nominal Rate Copies Mailed at Other Classes Through the USPS (e.g. First-Class Mail)		
	(4) Free or Nominal Rate Distribution Outside the Mail (Carriers or other means)		
e. Total Free or Nominal Rate Distribution (Sum of 15d (1), (2), (3) and (4)		40	46
f. Total Distribution (Sum of 15c and 15e) ►		906	818
g. Copies not Distributed (See instructions to publishers #4 (page #3)) ►		434	502
h. Total (Sum of 15f and g)		1340	1320
i. Percent Paid (15c divided by 15f times 100) ►		95.58%	94.38%

16. Publication of Statement of Ownership
    ☐ If the publication is a general publication, publication of this statement is required. Will be printed in the **December 2011** issue of this publication. ☐ Publication not required

17. Signature and Title of Editor, Publisher, Business Manager, or Owner

    Stephen R. Bushing –Inventory Distribution Coordinator

    Date: September 16, 2011

I certify that all information furnished on this form is true and complete. I understand that anyone who furnishes false or misleading information on this form or who omits material or information requested on the form may be subject to criminal sanctions (including fines and imprisonment) and/or civil sanctions (including civil penalties).

PS Form **3526**, September 2007 (Page 2 of 3)

Printed and bound by CPI Group (UK) Ltd, Croydon, CR0 4YY
03/10/2024
01040461-0018